Psychiatric Hospital Closure

'When someone died here, the bell used always to ring....
When it rung, everyone said: O, God, please let me die, as I
am tired of continuing this life inside this place.... There
was nothing to do, because they found themselves closed
here inside and had no hope of getting out. It is like a plant
fading because it did not rain and the leaves wither, this is
what people here were like'.

Andrea, in the Psychiatric Hospital of Gorizia,
L'istituzione Negata, Einaudi, Torin, 1, 1968.

Psychiatric Hospital Closure

Myths and realities

Edited by
Shulamit Ramon

Senior Lecturer
Social Work
and
Course Director
Mental Health Work with the Continued Care Client
London School of Economics
UK

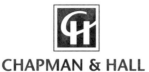

CHAPMAN & HALL

London · Glasgow · New York · Tokyo · Melbourne · Madras

Published by Chapman & Hall, 2–6 Boundary Row, London SE1 8HN

Chapman & Hall, 2–6 Boundary Row, London SE1 8HN, UK

Blackie Academic & Professional, Wester Cleddens Road, Bishopbriggs, Glasgow G64 2NZ, UK

Chapman & Hall, 29 West 35th Street, New York, NY10001, USA

Chapman & Hall Japan, Thomson Publishing Japan, Hirakawacho Nemoto Building, 7F, 1-7-11 Hirakawa-cho, Chiyoda-ku, Tokyo 102, Japan

Chapman & Hall Australia, Thomas Nelson Australia, 102 Dodds Street, South Melbourne, Victoria 3205, Australia

Chapman & Hall India, R. Seshadri, 32 Second Main Road, CIT East, Madras 600 035, India

Distributed in the USA and Canada by Singular Publishing Group Inc, 4284, 41st Street, San Diego, California 92105

First edition 1992

© 1992 Chapman & Hall

Typeset in 10/12 Palatino by EXPO Holdings, Petaling Jaya, Malaysia
Printed in Great Britain by T. J. Press, Padstow, Cornwall

ISBN 0 412 45000 3   1 56593 048 7 (USA)

A catalogue record for this book is available from the British Library

Library of Congress Cataloging-in-Publication data available

Contents

Contributors

Dr Christine McCourt-Perring is a Research Fellow at the Department of Government, Brunel University. An anthropologist by training, she is active in the Islington Forum.

Dr Shulamit Ramon is a Senior Lecturer in the Department of Social Administration, the London School of Economics — a social worker and clinical psychologist by training and author of: *Psychiatry in Britain: Meaning and Policy* (Croom Helm); editor and contributor to: *Psychiatry in Transition*: British and Italian Experiences (Pluto Press) and *Beyond Community Care*: Normalization and Integration Work (Macmillan).

Dr Dylan Tomlinson is Research Sociologist, Team for the Assessment of Psychiatric Services, North East Thames Health Region. He is a political scientist and sociologist by training and author of *Utopia, Community Care and the Retreat from the Asylums* (Open University Press).

Dr Tony Wainwright, Principal Psychologist, Camberwell and Maudsley Health Authority and Co-ordinator of the resettlement team of Cane Hill hospital. He is a clinical psychologist by training.

Acknowledgements

I would like to thank past and current residents and workers in psychiatric hospitals who have struggled with those institutions and thus have greatly contributed to our understanding of what needs to be improved in our mental health services and in our society.

The other contributors to this book have been generous in sharing their ideas, tolerant of my intrusion into their hectic schedules, and enthusiastic about the project to which they have brought considerable experience and knowledge, turning working together into an enjoyable experience for me. Jo Campling continued to offer advice and support whenever required, despite all of her other commitments.

Aelita suffered long weekends of maternal neglect with the genuine relish of a teenager and yet has developed an interest in mental health issues: I therefore dedicate this book to her.

Preface

A major British parliamentary committee on mental health services for adults commented in its report that 'any fool can close a hospital' (Social Services Committee, 1985). This book illustrates that even the wisest person would have found the task of closing a psychiatric hospital most complex and demanding, yet challenging and exhilarating at the same time. That this committee of eminent parliamentarians, which has listened carefully to the evidence of many witnesses and read a lot more on the subject matter, would thus conclude its deliberations, highlights the emphasis on services in the community to the point of being unable to focus on hospital closure in its own right, instead of being treated as an insignificant step towards a community mental health system.

A different message is proposed in this book. The text demonstrates how crucial is the **process** of hospital closure for both the outcomes of such closure, as well as for the future services in the community. In a number of ways future services are defined and planned as part of the resettlement component of hospital closure, a point illustrated time and again in each chapter of this book.

A British psychiatrist whose intelligence and knowledge I greatly value has recently reacted to a suggestion to focus on hospital closure in a professional journal by stating that this would have been relevant in the 1980s, but not in the 1990s. The lack of any research or current discussion as to what has happened in the massive closures of North American hospitals in the 1960s and the 1970s would indicate that, there too, professionals do not see such closures as related to their present services and their dilemmas. This book highlights that, unless we are able to understand the full impact of hospital closure on the direct and indirect participants in this endeavour, we as societies, countries, and people will be unable to connect our psychiatric past to our psychiatric present and future, and consequently unable to learn some most valuable lessons. Moreover, in many western countries the process of hospital closure has only started, with Second and Third World countries still aspiring to build large psychiatric hospitals. It would therefore seem that, far from being a matter of a long forgotten past, this is very much an issue of the present and of the future.

Although hospitals for people with learning difficulties have closed in western countries (Glennerster and Korman, 1990) and more are due to close in the near future, it is the closure of the **psychiatric hospitals** that has been perceived from the beginning as controversial, leading to a heated debate concerning the 'pros' and 'cons' of such a move.

This book contributes to this debate by attempting to explain the background for the closure, illustrating, through working examples, key issues and processes entailed in such closures and analysing the significance of what has happened as part of psychiatric hospitals closure.

We are all **stake holders** in this crucial process of restructuring our mental health systems, because it affects directly and indirectly all of us. Some of us find ourselves more centrally involved in this process, such as service users and their relatives, workers in mental health services, planners of the services and politicians. This book focuses on three out of these five stake holders, service users, workers, and planners, and references to the two others are made when relevant. Were we to include all stake holders, more than one volume would have become necessary.

The authors' own backgrounds reflect the different disciplines whose knowledge base is used for the purpose of a better understanding of the complex processes involved in exploring hospital closure: anthropology, psychology, sociology and social work. Their life experiences include being service users, workers, planners and researchers. The contributors do not necessarily share in full the same perspective on hospital closure, but they share the belief in its importance for the future of our mental health services and the belief in the need to approach the closure **as a partnership** that involves all of the different stake holders.

A number of specific instances of hospital closure are described in the book as case studies, to provide the reader with in-depth knowledge of what hospital closure entails for the different participants involved in it. At the same time, the wider implications of these specific situations are pointed out and related to the major conceptual and action-orientated issues.

No attempt has been made to gloss over the inevitable, and numerous, conflicts that hospital closure contains. To the contrary, these conflicts have been highlighted, together with the ways and means by which they have been handled and at times satisfactorily resolved, not only for the sake of telling the story as it was for its main actors, but aiming at exploring myths and realities from the different perspectives of the stakeholders. Myth is defined in the dictionary as 'a legend, a poetic fiction', or as 'a fabulous narrative founded on some event'. It is suggested here that the fears and hopes concerning the outcomes of psychiatric hospitals closure should be treated as myths because, while containing elements of reality, they are embroidered upon according to the fears and hopes derived from beliefs on mental distress and people who suffer from it, which in turn relate to individual and collective world views. This book is aimed at sorting out the basis for the fears and the hopes, as some fears and some hopes have a more sound base in reality, whereas others are indeed a 'fabulous narrative based on an event'.

I hope that the reader will not only gain information and knowledge from this book, but will also become involved with and intrigued by the unfolding stories and processes.

We believe that hospital closures can offer opportunities for a better future to all of the stakeholders. For that to happen the barriers that are candidly explored in this book are considered, together with suggestions as to the adequate steps that can be taken to overcome them, for a participative vision of mental health services in the community to have a better chance to materialize.

Shulamit Ramon
November 1991

REFERENCES

The Social Services Select Committee (1985) *Community Care, With Special References to Adult Mentally Ill and Mentally Handicapped People*, Vol. 1. London, HMSO.
Glennerster, H. and Korman, N. (1990) *Closing a Hospital*. Open University, Milton Keynes.

Introduction

Twenty years of our history have been returned to us
Vaclav Havel, May 1989, in Prague.

THE CONTEXT OF HOSPITAL CLOSURE IN THE WESTERN WORLD, OR WHY NOW?

The significance of closing psychiatric hospitals

Psychiatric hospitals have been with us in the Western World since the late eighteenth century as the major form of social and professional response to serious mental distress. Rothman (1971), when writing about the American hospitals, illustrated how much they were intended as offering a humane alternative to previous forms of intervention. The move to psychiatric hospitalization on a massive scale was part of perceiving madness as a disease that requires medical treatment, with hospitals as the site for the application of such a technology.

The belief in medical technology has increased in the twentieth century and general hospitals have become citadels of high technology. Yet, simultaneously, people with physical illness began to stay less in hospital and be treated more outside it. Since the 1950s, the same happened to people suffering from mental distress, even though the level of pure technology and the availability of **curing** medication (as opposed to arresting symptoms or reducing level of activity and suffering) has been much lower in relation to mental illness. The dramatic change in the pattern of hospitalization is best exemplified in statistics concerning its length throughout the Western World. Whereas, before World War II the majority of in-patients stayed for life in hospital (for 20–40 years!), this was reduced to ten years in the 1950s, and stands now at less than a month for 60% of the British in-patients and 80% of the Italian in-patients (Health and Personal Social Services Statistics (HPSSS) for England, 1990; Crepet, 1990).

However, in most Western countries, there are still groups of people who have been in hospital between five and 20 years. **Resettlement** has been primarily concerned with this long-stay population, as described in Chapters 1, 2 and 4. However, a much larger number comes and goes frequently into either psychiatric hospitals, psychiatric wards in general hospitals, or into closed facilities (the American term for units of up to 100 people who remain there for up to one year). Estimated at about 1 500 000 in the USA, and 150 000 in the UK (Hollingworth, 1990; Ramon, 1990), admitting them to hospital is rather expensive, at around £300–500 per person per week in 1991 in the UK (Knapp and Beecham, 1991), and the long-term value of hospitalization doubtful.

Motives for proposing closure

The call for the closure of psychiatric hospitals has come from more than one source, and has more than one motive. It dates from the 1950s and originated in the USA by psychiatrists who were involved in initiating the 'Open Door' policy there, namely having open wards and an early discharge policy. Their logic was that if it were possible to discharge people earlier from hospital, it should be possible to prevent admission by earlier and improved intervention in the community (Brown, 1985). They were ardent believers in the value of medical treatment, as well as in that of psychological intervention, and did not perceive these two approaches incompatible.

Their call was echoed and reinforced by two unlikely partners; politicians and sociologists. American politicians (and later Australian, British, Dutch, Italian and New Zealand politicians, to name some of the countries already implementing hospital closures) were attracted to the combination of a promised reduced public expenditure and a more respectful way of treating fellow citizens. As lay people, they were pleased to rely on professional advice, especially when that advice suited their financial and ideological preferences, such as the reliance on the use of the family (especially of female relatives) for unpaid labour, or the fascination with the ever-elastic concept of the community (Scull, 1978). They also did not (and still do not) doubt the value of medical contribution or the belief that mental illnesses were diseases, perceiving of care in the community as compatible with the achievements of psychiatrists (Ramon, 1985).

Across the Western World, sociologists with a growing interest in understanding the social roots of creating and maintaining deviant behaviour and identity have come to the conclusion that hospitals are social institutions that maintain people judged to suffer mental illness by segregating them as deviants from the rest of society. Goffman (1961) has contributed to this focus by comparing life in a psychiatric hospital with life in prison in terms of the regimentation, lack of choice and an imposed master status. Famous for coining the term **'total institution'** (which is expanded upon in Chapter 4), his work on **stigma** and internalized **deviant identity** is not less relevant to understanding a central element of the assumed impact of hospitalization and the afterlife of the patient-person (Goffman, 1963).

The concept of **de-institutionalization** by which the dual processes of dehospitalization and resettling in the community are often referred to comes from this focus. Following a long-honoured tradition of social psychologists and sociologists of knowledge (such as Durkhiem, Weber, Mead and Schutz), Becker, Garfinkel, Goffman, Lemert, Matza and Scheff (1975), among others, proposed that while many people indulge in breaking rules of normative behaviour, only a few are sufficiently unlucky to be caught in the process, notably (but not exclusively) when committing a crime. While it is natural for society to defend itself against criminal behaviour, this school of sociology argued that the zeal often demonstrated by society in segregating and stigmatizing individuals who committed crimes relates to enhancing the fear of the non-criminals of their own attraction to crime, rather than to deterring criminals from committing further offences.

On the surface, madness is very different from crime, in terms of intentionality, degree of rational control over one's action and physical harm done to others or to property. Nevertheless, these sociologists suggested that through the segregation in hospital and the ongoing stigma that continues to be attached after discharge, people who have exhibited madness are treated similarly to those who committed criminal offences in terms of the implications for their self and social images and roles.

Perhaps because the boundary between sanity and madness is so 'grey' the **social** boundary is felt as having to be so much more rigid, and the sanctions of crossing the threshold into madness so forceful and imposing, to prevent people from being threatened by the madness that potentially resides in all of us. Treating madness as a disease whose treatment requires segregation has been the symbol of these rigid boundaries, according to the sociology of deviance. Thus their approach focuses on the social construction of madness and views with scepticism being its medical perspective.

While proposed for a variety of motives, hospital closure nevertheless symbolizes the unifying wish to opt for a less segregated social attitude, of accepting that hospitals were a mistaken form of intervention, and of recognizing that there is a place for people who exhibit madness in our midst.

Finally, while the need and right of asylum is acceptable to all of us, the sight of so many people segregated from ordinary living has led to a sense of moral indignation especially among people who were hospitalized, relatives and friends, professionals, politicians and people of the media. **Moral outrage** has the power to make people fight for the abolition of unsatisfactory solutions and for the creation of better solutions (Robb, 1967; Cochrane, 1990).

Doubts and fears concerning closure

These relatively new ideas are not easily palatable for any of the participants in this drama, as they imply that:

1. A large number of people have unnecessarily spent many years away from ordinary living; have lost contacts, abilities, and ordinary life pleasures and achievements, largely irrevocably.
2. A large number of professional workers have unnecessarily spent their professional life in not providing the best available intervention, and in reinforcing the controlling element of their work instead of the caring element.
3. A huge amount of public money, and in some countries also private money, has been mis-spent.

4. Collective guilt has been building up, together with ambivalence towards people who exhibit madness, and unease and threat felt in relation to having them living next to us.
5. Relatives have felt let down by the rest of us, as the necessary alternatives to hospitalization have been slow to develop, and the rate of development has been uneven in different parts of each country. At the same time relatives are implicitly expected by politicians to be able to shoulder the responsibility for the suffering family member, without a parallel sufficient development in support services for the relatives, and without questioning the wisdom of such an imposition for all family members.
6. Fears of the re-creation of mini-institutions in the community, as a way of re-containing people with mental illness.
7. There is no professional or public consensus on what should replace the hospital as the core intervention unit and, consequently, there is no mobilization of people behind a well-structured approach, which attempts to meet head-on most of the fears and doubts.

The latter point is less surprising than it may seem, as it is easier to reach consensus on what is morally unacceptable than on what is acceptable, because the latter requires much more meticulous thought and investment. In relation to hospital closure, the complexity of meeting needs and supporting people when they leave hospital is combined with a lack of consensus as to the origins of mental illness and therefore as to what constitutes suitable intervention. This is coupled with ignorance of the available evaluated interventions because of: (a) not wanting to know about alternatives to hospitalization for a long time; (b) the complexity coming out of individual differences; and (c) the need to apply both individualized and group solutions to resettlement and to the prevention of chronicity.

Fears in the community of violence, bizarre behaviour and unkempt appearance that are expected of people labelled as mad coming to live near them, together with the mismatch between meeting needs and establishing services on time and inadequate financial resources or an inadequate use of these resources all add to the cocktail of the difficulties to reach a consensus, the lack of which has a 'snowball' effect.

Fear of homelessness and neglect in the community of resettled people, and even more so of those who have not responded as professionals expected to services on offer (namely the so-called non-compliant clients), is particularly voiced in any comparison between hospital and community services. This is based on the belief that the hospital offered shelter and asylum besides containment, and that these functions are not adequately offered without the brick-and-mortar effect of a building called a hospital. Thus the search for a new **symbolic,** yet **concrete,** site that will meet these sentiments is unfinished. Whether such a site could, or should, meet these functions is another matter. This issue is touched upon in all the chapters in this book on the value and application of the normalization (or social role valorization; SRV) approach to closure and resettlement processes.

The issue of the assumed drift into homelessness of people with mental illness when hospitals disappear deserves special attention as it highlights the view that these people are incapable of leading an ordinary life with support. There is extremely little evidence to support this assumption when housing is made available at an affordable cost to most people with mental illness. The evidence strongly suggests that they become homeless due to a fall-out in relations with those with whom they live. They are evicted, either when they are in a crisis and neglect the property, or to suit the financial interest of the house owners (Kay and Legg, 1985).

The minority that seems to become voluntarily homeless usually suffers from drink and drug misuse as well as mental illness, and is often also disillusioned with any formal service providers. What is striking in the current public debate on mental health services in Britain, Italy and the USA is the relative lack of vigour in defending hospitals or calling for their reinstatement, coupled with considerable scepticism that care in the community can work for people with serious mental health problems. This highlights the paucity of developing alternative models and/or of convincing the public that they are indeed workable alternatives.

Cost-effectiveness

There are fears that the cost of care in the community for the people leaving hospital will be more expensive than to keep them in hospital. Today such a consideration is taken very seriously, especially by governments and statutory service providers. There are very few comprehensive calculations that separate out the cost of looking after people in hospital, the initial cost of closing the hospital and resettling them in the community, and the more long-term costs. This is made all the more complex because within the hospital-leavers group there are a number of subgroups; there are also a number of subgroups among those who might have been hospitalized but who would not be, or at least not for long periods of time, and the differential costing has to take into account all of these variations. Furthermore, as hospitals are total institutions, residents were not using ordinary services available to all citizens, such as primary health care and libraries. Once they live in the community they are hopefully making use of these services, and therefore some economists argue that the cost of these components should be included too. This is an example of **indirect costs**, as these elements are not usually calculated for other citizens, even when they are receiving state benefits.

Existing accounts of closure and resettlement across different client groups are conflicting (Glennerster and Korman, 1990; Shiells and Wright, 1990). Detailed accounts of two British planned closure and resettlement schemes (three small hospitals in the Exeter district and the larger Friern

Barnet and Claybury hospitals in the North East Thames Health Region) illustrate that it is cheaper to keep a person even in a highly supportive setting in the community than in the hospital (King, 1991; Knapp and Beecham, 1990). Italian figures highlight that no decrease in overall spending takes place when hospitals close down (admittedly from a low level of spending in comparison with countries such as Britain) but that there is a **redistribution** in the proportion of money spent on different items of the budget. Thus less money is spent on capital investment in the community after the initial investment, less money is spent on medication, but more is paid to staff even though the number of workers has remained the same in the community as in the hospital (Mauri, 1986).

As only a minority requires very supportive resettlement, one subgroup of the most supported leavers is likely not to go on living for a long time due to old age (70+ years), and hopefully fewer people in the community will require long-term support when services in the community become fully operational, it would seem that hospitals remain the most expensive solution and care in the community is likely to be a cheaper option.

This assumption is further borne out by the reduction in cost after the initial set-up phase of some of the most comprehensive and long-term services, such as the TCL (Training in Community Living) in Madison, Wisconsin, and the London-based Daily Living Programme (Stein, 1990; Muijen, Marks and Connolly, 1990).

Hopes of hospital closure

The fears relate to beliefs in the fixed nature of mental illness and doubts as to the usefulness of existing interventions and resources. In turn, the hopes associated with hospital closure relate to beliefs in the positive ability of people to respond to improved conditions and ways of interacting with them, as well as to the wish to undo the harm created by years of segregation.

Throughout the Western World many small-scale initiatives that focused on the rehabilitation and re-integration of people with many years of hospitalization, and/or with a large number of short admissions, took place since the 1950s. The evaluated outcomes of these projects indicate cautious optimism concerning the prospects of people who are leaving the hospitals now, as well as outlining the need for **continuous** support to ensure positive results (Burti and Mosher, 1989; Hoult, 1986).

The known findings from large-scale closures are, on the whole, less systematically monitored, but indicate that, when the closure and the resettlement are planned, gradual and followed through, the majority of the hospital residents will do reasonably well in terms of no overall increase in clinical symptoms. As a result they have no need for hospitalization, a degree of self-care and social skills necessary for shared living, and a degree of subjective satisfaction. Some of them may relapse and a larger proportion than in the general population suffers from physical ill health. In those hospital closure and resettlement projects that emphasize social interaction in the community and employment, as in a number of Italian cities, the outcomes in relation to these areas are more encouraging than they are in projects that take for granted a highly sheltered, non-integrated existence. A link between **expectations** (by carers and by the residents themselves), opportunities, support, and **outcomes** is indicated.

Where attention has been paid to establishing easily accessible, non-medicalized, crisis refuge facilities, the evidence highlights a considerable reduction in the need for hospital admission to units in general hospitals. This also implies that it is possible to break the cycle of repeated short admissions and sliding into chronicity by investing in alternative asylum facilities in the community (Warner, 1991; Test *et al.*, 1985; Echlin and Ramon, 1992).

Even the minority group with a combination of mental illness, drink, drug misuse and homelessness responds to, and benefits from, the work of non-statutory, usually non-professional, carers. These carers offer a range of services from basic shelter and food, welfare rights and tribunal representation, to drop-in user-managed centres and, in some cases, to independent living schemes supported by professionals (Cheema, 1991).

The feared backlash by the public has not materialized in any country where hospitals have closed down and residents went to live in the community, perhaps because the feared violence by ex-patients did not take place in any substantial form. Where effort was made to secure a positive public reception this has resulted in a less indifferent, more friendly, attitude.

Likewise, where a concerted attempt to provide support for relatives has taken place, relatives' attitudes have been more positive towards hospital closure and resettlement.

The conceptual and moral basis for the hopes associated with closure and resettlement

Conceptually and morally the normalization/social role valorization (SRV) approach encapsulates best the hopes for the ex-residents of the psychiatric hospitals and for the future of the mental health services and their users.

Elements of this approach appear in particular in Chapters One and Four, as they relate to issues of what has been lost through prolonged hospitalization by hospital residents, and in the discussion of whether the forms of resettlement adopted for them constitute an ordinary life or not. Chapter Two illustrates the implications of a wide-ranging interpretation of the approach by people who, while largely uninformed about it, assume that the approach is so commonsensical that there is no need to become better informed.

The SRV approach takes from the deviancy approach in sociology the belief in the importance of self-image and the image fostered on us by the way others views us. Applying it to people with disability, SRV theorists argue that this group of people is devalued, as the social definition of the disability will prevent people who suffer from it from fulfilling valued roles in society, from contributing to the life of others, and from being able to look after themselves. Elsewhere I have suggested that they suffer from the impact of a double act of devaluation, perceived to be different in a negative sense, have been segregated on this basis, have been prevented from taking on valued roles, and are consequently further devalued as unable to perform these roles (Ramon, 1991).

Instead, it is suggested that this set of beliefs is not only morally repugnant, but unjustified in terms of what these people can contribute now and in terms of what they would be able to contribute were they not put in a devalued, totally other-dependent position for a long time (Wolfensberger, 1983). Their ability to contribute stems from the fact that the disability is **only one** of their characteristics and, in common with all other human beings, they too have positive and negative qualities, abilities and deficiencies. In addition, it is argued that the disability to perform and to use one's own positive abilities is linked to the imposition of dependency and irresponsibility within any form of institutionalized living. Stripped out of such a setting, people can regain their dignity, sense of responsibility, and ability to function at a higher level than previously, provided they are given the right opportunities and non-patronizing support.

For this shift to happen there is a need for a parallel shift in removing the barriers that they face, and in a considerable attitudinal change among all of us. If the person with a disability has to change his/her self-image and ways of relating to others, relatives have to enable the person to take responsibility, to take risks, to be involved in their socially valued activities, and not to be treated as incapable of doing so because of the disability. Professionals too have to realize that they do not necessarily know best (even if sometime they may indeed know best), and that 'their' clients should be encouraged to take calculated risks as part of the path towards a greater sense of self and social worth. Professionals have to be enablers as much as possible and if they need to do things for a person this has to be negotiated with that person, and has to be as specific and as minimal as possible. A good example of this approach is provided by the brokerage model, in which the client is the employer of the people who provide him/her with an agreed package of services that has been negotiated with the client and other relevant people, even if the source of the money to pay the broker and the service givers may come from the state or the local authority (Brandon and Towe, 1990). In this example, power relations have shifted, with the client getting more power and a greater measure of control over his/her life, while the traditional service providers give up at least some of their power.

Thus the normalization approach firmly advocates not only a model of citizens' equality and right to services but also a greater degree of power to service users. This is further exemplified in the focus on the evaluation of services by users and by staff from the perspective of providing a non-stigmatizing, enabling service at every aspect of the service. (See the PASS approach, referred to in Chapter One and by Glenn and Wolfensberger (1973), and for its application to a British day hospital, Wainwright *et al.* (1988).)

The approach originated in the field of learning difficulties, and then expanded to people with physical disabilities. Most of the attempts to apply it have been in relation to the first two areas, and the evidence of success in enhancing people's quality of life has been impressive. This way of thinking does not set out to be cost-effective, as the quality of service and opportunities are of paramount importance.

The reader may well ask if this approach is equally relevant to the field of mental illness, and to people who suffer from it. This question can be asked by those who believe in the disease model of mental illness, as much as by those who see mental distress not as a disability but a response to problems of living. The SRV approach does not take a position as to whether mental distress is a disease, an illness, or a long-term impairment, but assumes that people who have suffered from it have been segregated and devalued, and focuses on this dimension to the exclusion of consideration of the origins of mental distress. Thus a belief in the biological origin of mental illness can be accommodated within this approach so long as this does not carry with it the assumption that the person is unable to benefit from ordinary living and has the capacity to contribute to some aspects of such a living. Likewise, the SRV stance can accommodate the perspective of problems in living if it is accepted that the implications of suffering from these problems also imply not only being devalued by others, but by oneself, as well as having to overcome internalized and external pressure, and not be responsible and not to contribute to the life of others and oneself in an active way.

In short, within the SRV framework the existence of disabilities is accepted, and no interest is expressed in attributing blame for the initial source of the disability or for finding its origins. Instead the focus is on how best to live with the handicap or overcome it if possible. When extended to mental distress, especially to people who are in hospital or have been hospitalized for long periods, the approach has far-reaching conceptual and empirical consequences. It leads to a different way of assessment (Chapter One), a different way of looking at medical files and people's past history (Chapter Four), a different vision of the process of dehospitalization and of the role of the professionals (Chapter Three) and of that of resettlement (Chapters One, Two and Four).

The aim of the above description of the normalization school of thought is neither to provide a comprehensive presentation of it nor to suggest that it does not have its own shortcomings or problems. It is only to relate this framework to hospital closure and resettlement. Like most developing approaches, there is more than one strand to it, and there are disagreements and contradictions among the different protagonists. The reader interested in further information on the approach can look at the papers by Wolfensberger (1972), Tyne and O'Brien (1981), Wainwright *et al.* (1988), Brandon (1991) and Ramon (1991).

Criticisms against the SRV approach

The main criticisms levelled against this approach that the reader should consider are that it: (a) is widely optimistic and over-demanding from clients and society; (b) imposes a North American middle-class style of living on everyone; and (c) may lead to the exploitation of informal carers (the majority of whom are women) in the name of the right of users to lead an ordinary life. As with every conceptual and practice-orientated approach, the reader is invited to take an **irreverent** attitude to this specific framework, and to all others.

Emerging partners

Users' involvement and user-managed services

This is a recent development, more prevalent in a formalized way in Holland, North America, Britain and Australia than in other countries. It is not unlinked to the SRV approach and to the focus on citizens rights, especially that of ethnic minorities, women and gay people, since the 1960s. Part of the new wave of social movements (Toch, 1965), collective users' groups have also developed in response to recent critique of the impersonal character of the welfare state (Offe, 1984) and of professional power (Chamberlin, 1979). Rogers and Pilgrim (1991) provide an interesting account of the development of the British movement where several of these components have been expressed.

Users' participation is based on the view that the users' perspective on their difficulties and on services offered to them is as valid as that of the other participants in their scenario, and has to be taken into account in any consideration of what will happen to them individually and collectively, that is in planning and evaluating services too. As such, it represents a considerable shift from the perspective of the mad person as the carrier of a disease or of pathological features that distort his/her perception to the point that it cannot be treated as valid. Instead, it is suggested that, while some aspects of the person's behaviour and experience may indeed be mad, the person has nevertheless a useful insight into his/her plight and the interventions that might be helpful or unhelpful to him/her. This per-spective emphasizes that the mad component of the person is not all of what there is to the person, and that other qualities and abilities should be encouraged and taken into account in any decision-making processes concerning the person. At the collective level, this position implies that users should be consulted properly and listened to regarding policies and services on the one hand, and in the more fundamental rethinking as to what is madness about.

Given that many users of mental health services have been critical of what the services offer, the adoption of the users' perspective implies also a tacit acceptance that there is room for criticism and improvement in this field.

The available forms of users' involvement are as follows:

1. *Patients' councils* in hospitals and outside, which focus on encouraging patients to express their views on any issue related to their situation, providing information and access into self and peer advocacy (in Holland and some British towns).
2. *Users' forums* in neighbourhoods in which people share information and views, and act as policy formation and pressure groups, as well as a mutual support network (in Britain, USA, Canada);
3. Users' own *advocacy schemes* (in Holland, Britain and USA);
4. Users as *members* of mental health services *management committees* (in UK and USA).
5. Users as *evaluators* of service provision (in Britain, Canada and USA);
6. Users as *researchers* (in USA);
7. Users as service *providers*, either within a service that includes other carers, or in services only manned by users (Australia, Britain, USA and Holland).
8. Users as organizers and participants in *mutual* (self) *help* groups (everywhere).

Although most of the activists in users' groups operate from the community, they tend to come from among those who have been hospitalized, often after repeated and prolonged periods of hospitalization. Nearly all known users' groups welcome the closure of psychiatric hospitals, as they have been consistently critical of hospitalization as a helpful intervention, instead viewing it as an abusive environment in more than one aspect of living (Lawson, 1991). Some groups have developed befriending schemes for hospital residents, proposed a better code for admissions, and established the patients' councils within the hospital wards (Nottingham Advocacy Group, 1989).

Relatives' involvement

Relatives have been always involved as individuals, and some of them as benefactors or initiators of support systems for people with mental illness. However, since the 1970s relatives' organizations have been developing in many Western countries, such as Britain, Italy, the Scandinavian countries, and the USA. In contrast to users' groups, there is less variety in how these groups are organized, what they provide to members, and what they stand for. They are organized as mutual support and campaigning groups both nationally and locally, which have become more numerous and gained momentum in direct relation to hospital closure. Most groups oppose this policy strongly and advocate the re-opening of hospitals, establishing special units for people with long-term mental health difficulties, or the prevention of hospital closure (Weleminsky, 1990).

Where national organizations exist (e.g. in the USA and UK), they have considerable political clout and financial resources at their disposal, unlike the users' groups. This is understandable as there are no doubts concerning their sanity, their suffering attracts sympathy easily as it is not 'tainted' with the suspicion of either madness or badness, and their view of mental illness as a disease echoes dominant professional views and those of the general public (Hatfield, 1987).

Given this background, it is, in fact, surprising that they are yet to have a more significant impact on policies in any country. This is perhaps due to the lack of alternatives in their presentations to what exists but is found wanting for a variety of reasons. This could also reflect on the general indifference towards mental illness and people associated with it, together with fear, fascination and the wish to distance oneself from anything or anybody related to it.

The lack of congruency, or the open conflict that often manifests itself between users and relatives, weakens the pressure power of both groups. Therefore it would have been preferable if they could unite in their position on key issues, such as the need for housing and income. However, to suggest an artificial unity for the sake of campaigning together would be inappropriate and misleading.

Care staff

There were always unqualified care staff working in mental health services, but their number has increased considerably with the closure of hospitals. They are to be found especially in residential and day-care facilities, where many of the continuing-care clients congregate. Home-helps, brokers, some community support workers and care managers are among the more recent participants in this staff group. Their position is ambiguous, and so it would seem is their self-image. They are providing a needed service and are expected to conform to a professional code of behaviour and service standard, yet they have not been trained specifically to do so. Likewise, their salaries tend to be much lower than that of qualified staff, even when their responsibilities are not.

The issues of the relationships between professionally qualified and un-qualified care staff, the usefulness of each group to service users and relatives, the social status of this group all await the serious debate that they deserve. Chapter Four illustrates vividly these issues in the closure situation.

The non-statutory sector

In many Western countries there are two types of non-statutory organizations active in the field of mental health, namely non-profit (the voluntary sector in Britain) and for-profit agencies. While the first group has been usually acting as a pressure group and, at times, in a service-providing capacity, the second has been involved only in service provision.

Traditionally the non-profit organizations have also been more innovative and liberal-minded in their approach to people with mental illness than either the statutory sector or the for-profit organizations. Hospitals tended to be part of the statutory sector or the for-profit subsector, while services in the community were developed by the non-profit sector throughout the Western World.

In the cold welfare climate that is still with us since the mid-1970s, governments have been attempting to encourage the expansion of the non-statutory sector, perceiving this to be more economical and less centralized. Indeed, this expansion has taken place.

Concerning the for-profit subsector, a much cheaper service that competes financially with the statutory provided services has emerged, with little to show in quality. In fact, in many cases service quality is considerably lower than in either the statutory or the non-profit sectors. Furthermore, the for-profit subsector has been uninterested in generating a comprehensive service, and has concentrated on the sections that provide handsome profit, moving from one service to another, in accordance to the profit margin.

In contrast, the non-profit subsector has provided a cheaper service, often of good quality, and at times innovative, in an area of service where neither the statutory nor the for-profit group were inclined to invest. Appendix A illustrates how these emerging partners operate within the policy and practice context of one society, namely Britain.

The mental health service systems of most Western countries are undergoing a far-reaching change, in which many 'taken-for-granted' beliefs are questioned, in particular the centrality of psychiatric hospitals within these systems. While I am unable to predict the final outcomes of this change, I feel privileged to be part of it, yet fearing the implications of some of its manifestations.

I hope that the readers will find this book to be a useful and challenging tool for their partnership within this crucial process of change.

REFERENCES

Brandon, D. and Towe, P. (1990) *Brokerage*. Good Impressions, London.

Brandon, D. (1991) *Innovation Without Change?* Macmillan, London.

Brown, P. (1985) *The Transfer of Care*. Routledge, London.

Burti, L. and Mosher, L. (eds) (1989) *Community Mental Health: Principles and Practice*. Norton, New York.

Chamberlin, J. (1979) *On Our Own*. McGraw-Hill, New York.

Cheema, B. (1991) *Berkeley and Oakland, Support Services*, Berkeley.

Cochrane, D. (1990) *The AEGIS Campaign to Improve Standards of Care in Hospitals: A Case Study of the Process of Social Policy Change*. PhD Thesis, London School of Economics.

Crepet, P. (1990) A transition period in psychiatric care in Italy: Ten years after the reform. *British Journal of Psychiatry*, **156**, 27–38.

Echlin, R. and Ramon, S. (1991) Alternative asylum in the community, *Nursing Times*, January 15th, 15–17.

Glenn, T. and Wolfensberger, W. (1973) *Programme Analysis of Service Systems (PASS): A Method for the Quantitative Analysis of Human Services*. Handbook of the National Institute on Mental Retardation, Toronto.

Glennerster, H. and Korman, N. (1990) *Closing a Hospital*. The Open University, Milton Keynes.

Goffman, I. (1961) *Asylums*. Penguin, Harmondsworth.

Goffman, I. (1963) *Stigma*. Penguin, Harmondsworth.

Hatfield, A. (1987) The National Alliance for the Mentally Ill: The meaning of a movement, *International Journal of Mental Health*, **15(4)**, 79–93.

Health and Personal Social Services Statistics (1990). HMSO, London.

Hollingworth, E.J. (1990) *Services in the Community for the Chronically Mentally Ill*. Conference on the division of labour in the health sector, Koln, Max Planck Institute, November 20th.

Hoult, J. (1986) Community care of the acutely mentally ill, *British Journal of Psychiatry*, **149**, 137–44.

Kay, A. and Legg, C. (1985) *Discharged to the Community: A Review of Housing and Support in London for People Leaving Psychiatric Care*. City University, London.

King, D. (1991) Replacing mental hospitals with better services. In: Ramon, S. (ed.) *Psychiatry in Transition*. Pluto Press, London.

Knapp, M. and Beecham, J. (1990) *Predicting the Community Costs of Closing Psychiatric Hospitals*. PSRRU, University of Kent, Canterbury.

Lawson, M (1991) A recipient's view In: Ramon, S. (ed.) *Beyond Community Care: Normalization and Integration Work*. Macmillan, London.

Mangen, S. (ed.) (1985) *Mental Health Care in the European Community*. Croom Helm, London.

Mauri, D. (1986) *La Liberta e Terapeuta?* Feltrinelli, Milano.

Muijen, M., Marks, I. and Connolly, J. (1990) The daily living programme: a controlled study of community care for the severely mentally ill in Camberwell. In: Hall, P. and Brockington, I. (ed.) *The Closure of Mental Hospitals*. Gaskell, London.

Nottingham Advocacy Group (1989) *Patients' Councils*, NAG, Nottingham.

Offe, C. (1984) *Contradictions of the Welfare State*. Hutchinson, London.

Ramon, S. (1985) *Psychiatry in Britain: Meaning and Policy*. Croom Helm, London.

Ramon, S. (1990) *Community Mental Health Services for the Continuing-Care Client*. Conference on the division of Labour in the Health Sector, Koln. Max Planck Institute, November 20th.

Ramon, S. (1991) Principles and conceptual knowledge. In: Ramon. S. (ed.) *Beyond Community Care: Normalization and Integration Work*. Macmillan, London.

Robb, B. (1967) *Sans Everything: A Case to Answer*. Nelson, London.

Rogers, A. and Pilgrim, D. (1991) Pulling down churches: accounting for the British Mental Health Users' Movement, *Sociology of Health and Illness*, **13 (2)**, 129–47.

Rothman, D. (1971) *The Discovery of the Asylum*. Little, Brown, Boston.

Scheff, T. (ed.) *Labelling Madness*. Prentice Hall, Englewood Cliffs, New Jersey.

Scull, A. (1978) *Decarceration*. Prentice Hall, Englewood Cliffs, New Jersey.

Shiells, A. and Wright, K. (1990) The economic costs. In: Alaszewski, A. and B.N. Ong, (eds) *Normalization in Practice*. Tavistock, London.

Stein, L. (1990) A systems approach to the treatment of people with chronic mental illness. In: Hall, P. and Brockington, I. (eds) *The Closure of Mental Hospitals*. Gaskell, London.

Test, M. A., Knoedler, W. H. and Allness, D. J. (1985) The long-term treatment of young schizophrenics in a community support programme. In: Stein, L. and Test, M.A. (eds.) *The Training in Community Living Model: A Decade of Experience, New Directions for Mental Health Service 26.* Jossey-Bass, San Francisco.

Toch, H. (1965) *The Social Psychology of Social Movements.* Bobbs Merrill, New York.

Tyne, A. and O'Brien, J. (1981) *The Principle of Normalization: A Foundation for Effective Services.* Campaign for Mental Handicap, London.

Wainwright, T., Holloway, F. and Brugha, T. (1988) Day care in an inner city. In: Lavender, A. and Holloway, F. (eds) *Community Care in Practice: Services for the Continuing-care Client.* Wiley, Chichester.

Warner, R. (1991) Creative programming. In: Ramon, S. (ed.) *Beyond Community Care: Normalization and Integration Work.* Macmillan, London.

Weleminsky, J. (1990) Contribution to the debate: This house recognizes the continued need for asylum. In: Hall, P. and Brockington, I. (eds.) *The Closure of Mental Hospitals.* Gaskell, London.

Wolfensberger, W. (1972) *The Principle of Normalization in Human Services.* National Institute of Mental Retardation, Toronto.

Wolfensberger, W. (1983) Social role valorization: a proposed new term for the principle of normalization, *Mental Retardation,* **21**, 234–9.

Part One
The Experience of Planning

Frequently, we or the systems which employ us do not and cannot treat those distressed people as if they were our neighbours, our brothers and sisters, our mothers and fathers. Until we do, and have structures which both support and encourage, innovation without change will continue.

David Brandon, 1991

The changing perspective of a resettlement team

TONY WAINWRIGHT

INTRODUCTION

This chapter describes the closure of Cane Hill Hospital, a large Victorian asylum, from the perspective of one member of the Camberwell Resettlement Team (CRT), which came into the hospital as part of the closure process. The team was employed by one of the District Health Authorities that had patients in the hospital. This chapter is not the result of a research study, but an account of my experience, which started in early 1984 and continues at the time of writing, when Cane Hill Hospital was due to close in six months time (October 1991). I have drawn heavily on the documents that were produced in great abundance during the last five years to illustrate the thinking that went on at different stages.

This chapter is divided into the following sections:

1. A historical introduction. This history is significant for two main reasons. Firstly, for the people who live and work in the hospital, this context contains one component of **their** history as some of them have lived and worked there for decades. Secondly, I believe that the relationships between the different agencies involved in the closure process were affected profoundly by the legends and myths about each other, the roots of which are buried in this historical context;
2. The establishment of the CRT and its work in developing a strategy and then setting up the framework for the new services, for example the staffed houses, the social club and work programmes, in a service environment of daunting complexity;
3. The work the CRT carried out in the hospital setting, including the problems we faced as outsiders welcomed into an institution with its own values and mores and actively promoting that same institution's demise. In addition, it will cover the work done in setting up the services, assisting the residents to move out and placement work;
4. Camberwell service developments and how they were implemented, including the work project, the cafe/social club and the advocacy service; and

5. A review of the way the process was managed and any lessons that may be learned.

HISTORICAL CONTEXT

The development of the South East Thames Regional Health Authority approach to hospital closure

Cane Hill Hospital is located in Coulsdon in Surrey, in the South East Thames Region and managed by Bromley Health Authority. The authority that owns the hospital is the South East Thames Regional Health Authority, and it was they who decided to close it as part of their wider objectives. Things proceeded slowly in the mental health field but, following the introduction of the NHS planning system in 1976, the Region set up a multi-disciplinary steering group to prepare strategies for the various client groups including the mentally ill. In 1985, their mental health strategy was published. This emphasized the importance of community care and set the tone, if not the details, of subsequent developments. The plans for hospital closures resulted in the policy statement '*A Service in Transition: Priorities for the Development of Local Mental Health Services to Replace Large Mental Hospitals in the South East Thames Region*' (1987).

Thus the closure of Cane Hill Hospital became top priority on the basis of seven dimensions, varying from estimates of the quality of the existing services to the robustness of the plans proposed by Districts. Locally, it had been anticipated for three years that Cane Hill would be closing, and the delay by the Region to confirm the closure led to considerable problems to involve the local authorities, who could not act until they had formal notice. On these dimensions Cane Hill scored top marks. In broad terms, this meant that at that time its existing services were poor (compared with the other six mental hospitals), the District plans were therefore reasonable, and the three Districts involved were committed to closure. However, it was significant that the level of Local Authority commitment and the personnel policy were identified as being poor, both issues that proved problematic.

The report also acknowledged that there would be high capital and revenue consequences but essentially committed the Region to the closure, relying on the possibility of large profits from selling the land on which the hospitals were built. Land sales during the period of the rapid price inflation of the earlier part of the 1980s had successfully funded some of the services that had replaced the mental handicap hospitals and homelessness institutions. It may have appeared at the time the strategy was developed, with talk of the economic miracle of 'Thatcherism', that land would continue to be saleable at vast profits. In the event, the value of the land was much less than anticipated and the funding has been severely squeezed in consequence. The anticipated timetable for closure was four years, and funding mechanisms were to be set up (for example the Mental Health Development Fund) to facilitate the process. The Region's subsequent involvement was in steering the process and, it seemed from time to time, changing the funding arrangements to keep us on our toes!

The history of Cane Hill Hospital

The beginnings of Cane Hill Hospital lie in the latter part of last century. The hospital has a carved stone block above the entrance inscribed with the date 1882, although the first patients were not transferred there until December 4th 1883 (Walk, 1952). It was the third mental hospital for the County of Surrey, which also had Springfield and Brookwood Hospitals, built over half a century earlier. During the 1850s and 1860s, these became very overcrowded and it was decided in 1875 that Cane Hill was needed. Financial matters also played a major role then (as now):

'...hundreds [of patients] had to be maintained in private asylums ('licensed houses') who made exorbitant charges on the Unions, which had lately been unreasonably raised. There were also many other patients living with their friends, who were not receiving adequate care.'

(Walk, 1952)

In another paper, Walk also makes the observation that:

...it is fairly clear that Cane Hill was founded really to save money and cut down the cost of admitting people to expensive private institutions.

(Walk, 1982)

Whether this was a general state of affairs or not is unclear.

In some counties, for example Cornwall (Andrews, 1978), there were concerns that the cost of housing people in the asylum would be heavier than keeping them in the workhouse, and so it was to prove. The Cornwall County Asylum Committee had to go to great lengths to keep their costs down in order to attract custom from the parishes. In order that their institution should be viable, they had to have an increasing number of paying customers. At one point, they invented a grade of patient, the so-called rate-aided patient, who paid more than the pauper but less than the private patient. This system afforded no better care than for the pauper, but reduced the stigma (Andrews, 1978). When the hospital was in its early stages of development, it was regarded as providing model treatment, and may have been used as the plan for other similar hospitals elsewhere. Early visitors were impressed with the way it was run. For example, the Commissioners in Lunacy (the pre-1913 inspection body) reported shortly after the opening of the hospital:

'The asylum is constructed for 1124 patients, 644 of the female, and 480 of the male sex. ...In the female division there are eight blocks... and in the male *six… [there] are the infirmaries… [blocks for] epileptic patients, [for] the suicidal, [for the] acute cases, the rest of the blocks are for the quiet and working patients. There is a detached hospital for infectious disorders, which is at present occupied by 11 women under the charge of a married attendant, and who cook and wash for themselves, and engage in needlework. …We find the wards well furnished and cheerful, and the substantial comfort of the patients fully secured.'*

(Commissioners in Lunacy, 1885)

It would appear that this honeymoon period did not last as it became increasingly overcrowded. Thus by 1889 it had been decided to build extensions, and numbers increased steadily until 1954 when they had reached peak of 2400. Since then, in parallel with national trends, the numbers have declined to just over 600 by 1985 and to less than 200 by April 1991 (Fig. 1.1). Although it clearly started well, the hospital had for many years been under-funded, even by comparison with other mental hospitals.

The revenue funding of Cane Hill has for many years compared unfavourably with all but a few large hospitals nationally. In 1983 the expenditure per in-patient day was recorded as £24.88. Within the South East Thames Region this compared with £30.15 at Bexley and £38.42 at Hellingly. In a survey of 180 mental-illness hospitals in that year, only five indicated lower figures. This impression is borne out by the so-called 'Yates indicators', which identify factors that may make a hospital 'at risk' compared with other hospitals. Cane

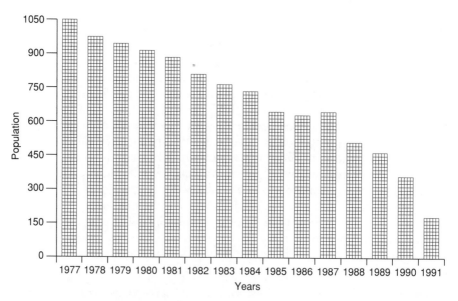

Figure 1.1   Patient population of Cane Hill Hospital between 1977 and 1991. (The populations in the years 1984 and 1990 were estimated.)

Hill performs poorly on three out of six indicators; the percentage of patients over 65, the number of patients per nurse and the length of stay of patients. Overall the analysis [...] in the S. E. Thames RHA's 'Regional Mental Health Strategy 1985–1994' concluded that Cane Hill was 'at risk'.

(Clifford, 1986)

This lack of resources was translated into very poor care practices. This is described in a report of an interview with the retiring director of nursing, Mr P. Philand.

'When Phil Philand went there as deputy chief male nurse in 1967 he found a regime which, in retrospect he says, seems 'unbelievable'. Patients were robbed of all dignity by practices rooted in the 19th-century attitudes to the mentally ill. Few kept personal possessions. None had their own clothing. Instead they shared clothes from a communal pool with other patients. All were kept under lock and key and had no privacy to wash or dress. And the sexes were kept strictly apart.'

(Purley and Coulsdon News, May 6th, 1988)

This is echoed in the Hospital Advisory Service (HAS) report on a visit in 1978:

'The intention to 'run-down' this very large and elderly establishment has been known and discussed over several years. The fulfilment of this intention is dependent on many eventualities, and as a result uncertainty has become endemic among the nurses employed in the hospital. This has been accentuated in recent years by the decline in patient numbers, and resulting in an increase in under-used wards and departments. It is not therefore a matter for surprise that the team was told repeatedly of lowered nursing morale, and of an under-current of dissatisfaction. There seem to have been few effective moves to inform nurses of the Area's intention for the future and the present situation is a frustrating and unsatisfactory one for the nurses. The general standard of nursing care is best described as benignly custodial, with a few wards showing a noticeably higher level of attainment.'

(HAS Report, 1978)

That the hospital population was running down is shown in Figure 1.1. From the peak occupancy of 2400 people in 1954, since 1977 the numbers have dropped from over 1000 to less than 200 at the time of writing.

Concerning physical standards of the hospital the HAS had this to say:

'The shop area is unattractive and squalid. The counter and displays are limited and insufficient for the numbers of patients, visitors and staff using the premises. The sales counter is situated at the narrow end of a large room. The whole room appears to serve two purposes: (a) as a sitting area and (b) as a shop supplying a limited range of goods. As a sitting area it is uninviting. With undefined cleaning arrangements the whole room is neglected, dirty and shabby.'

My first visit was in June 1986 with a colleague from Camberwell and I recorded some thoughts.

> 'We saw the OT department where there was an educational class like one might see in a Third World country, which appeared to be some sort of quiz. A solitary man was painting. The person conducting the quiz did not appear to be qualified. We found another place with Occupational Therapy on the door with a pleasant atmosphere. There were a number of women sitting doing knitting. A woman in a white coat seemed to be in charge. I asked if she was an Occupational Therapist and she said 'sort of'. She said she took all the patients the Occupational Therapy department didn't want. The place had a curiously empty feel. The wards we went to in the morning had crowded day rooms with inert people looking at television.'

The afternoon of that day we discussed the situation the hospital was in with one of the senior nursing staff.

> 'He said that one of the factors that was affecting progress at present was the belief among staff that they may lose their jobs if the place closes quickly.'[1]

Of the wards visited I noted:

> 'There was a lack of privacy. The men's ward was most depressing with many old men lying on their beds looking quite demoralized. The charge nurse seemed very lonely...'

The feelings among the staff were quite striking. On this first day we met with a charge nurse who burst into tears on telling us that she had learned that week that she and her husband would not be able to keep their home on the hospital campus. They had moved to the hospital in large measure as they understood they **could** keep it.

I also spent a day in the units providing activities for the patients and joined in as a participant, making these notes later.

> 'For the people living there life is impoverished. They have very low incomes and the hospital provides services at a rate per head among the lowest in the country. The available activities, although run by staff who, despite every-thing, maintain remarkable enthusiasm, are extremely limited. An example is the Nightingale Resocialization Unit. This is open daily during the week and is run by nurses and provides a place where people can go and engage in various games and other activities. While it certainly is welcomed by many patients as a pleasant place to go, and treats them with respect, the impression of an infant school atmosphere is striking. Such things as playing 'pass the parcel', shaking bottles filled with rice, and sticking cut-out pieces of maga-

---

[1] There were similar problems in Camberwell where St Giles Hospital, where I was based, and Dulwich North Hospital, where I also worked, were in the process of closing. Most of St Giles Hospital has since been demolished to make way for an expensive housing development. Dulwich is due to close in late 1991 or early 1992.

zine. Patients are given limited responsibility, a luxury in the hospital setting, and the staff report that many patients are remarkably more able in their setting than, for example, on the wards. Another example is the 'Pop-In'. Run by the Recreational Therapist (a qualified charge nurse) who by a remarkable series of initiatives has developed one of the most valuable hospital services, the Pop-In is a cafe on site, which also has an area for such things as social-skill training available. The recreational therapist also organizes many group outings, and has been helping the patients get to know something of the areas they will be returning to.'

(Wainwright, 1986)

So my first impressions of the staff in the hospital were mixed. Some people were very committed and skilled with what amounted to a calling for this work and who had strong personal relationships with the patients, but some staff were very demoralized. There were activities that ranged from those that were quite relevant to the patients needs to pretty appalling practices.

The staff's feelings about the closure of the hospital and our role in it were rarely expressed directly but, on one occasion, comment was passed that the resettlement teams were like maggots feasting on the entrails of a dying horse. This may convey something of the intensity of the feelings involved. A final graphic commentary on the state of feelings in the hospital was the cartoon found on the floor of one corridor (Figure 1.2).

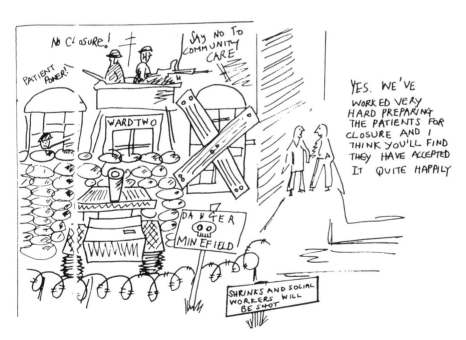

Figure 1.2 Cartoon found on the floor of one corridor in Cane Hill Hospital after the disclosure that the hospital was closing.

*The history of mental health services in the Camberwell Health District
and their relationship to Cane Hill*

A stable pattern of service provision involving Cane Hill developed after
World War I, when King's College Hospital and the Maudsley Hospital
became operational on their present sites. The other elements in the psychiatric hospital-type provision from that time included the Constance
Road Institution (which became St Francis' Hospital and is now known as
Dulwich North Hospital), a workhouse with psychiatric wards and the
Gordon Road Institution (later known as the Camberwell Reception
Centre), a workhouse for homeless men. This structure was in place by 1924
and, at that time, the pathway for a person who became mentally ill would
have been to have been admitted to the Constance Road Institution either
via a court order, or from the Gordon Road site. From here a decision
would have been made whether to route the patient to Cane Hill Hospital
or to the Maudsley Hospital. As noted by Isaacs and Bennett (1972) this
procedure became formalized.

> '...a pattern of care was set which continued for thirty-five years. The quiet
> voluntary 'patient' went to the Maudsley while St Francis received the
> objecting and objectionable but curable 'cases' and the mental hospitals took
> the 'chronics'...

The other element in the system was King's College Hospital's Department
of Psychological Medicine. King's College Hospital had a Chair of Psychological Medicine since 1871, and the emphasis of the department appears to
have been on the treatment of neurotic disorders, rather than the severe
mental health problems with which Cane Hill Hospital was being asked to
cope.

Camberwell's mental health services were divided into two since 1974,
when the Maudsley Hospital took the old parish of Camberwell as its
catchment area (now South Southwark). Camberwell Health Authority
provided for the rest, that is the East Lambeth sector via Cane Hill Hospital,
King's College Hospital and, progressively, via developing local services.
Cane Hill had established out-patient facilities in Camberwell in St Giles
Hospital in 1948, followed by acute inpatient wards there in 1972. A Day
Hospital on the same site opened in 1974. All these were seen at that time to
be part of the move to develop local services so that the District could stop
sending people to Cane Hill. The Maudsley Hospital ceased using Cane
Hill for general psychiatry in 1977, opening a local hostel and a variety of
work and day activities in its well-known District Services Centre.

The highly complex nature of this service network is significant in that it
provides some explanation for the stance that was taken by Cane Hill
Hospital, and by the Camberwell services during the closure process. Historical antagonisms were acted out at committee meetings, where it some-

times appeared that the players were consciously or unconsciously taking revenge on old enemies (as a result of past hurts) of the institutions they now represented. In 1984, when I first became involved with Cane Hill and its closure, Camberwell Health Authority had beds in the hospital for acute mental health problems, some long-stay beds and some beds for elderly people with dementia. In addition, the Maudsley Hospital had beds for elderly people with dementia. The Camberwell/Maudsley consultants who worked at the hospital also had beds in the local catchment area. The majority of the patients at this time were on the long-stay wards, and all were under the care of Bromley consultants and were very poorly known to the Camberwell services. The CRT's work would primarily be concentrated on the patients on the long-stay wards, and this lack of knowledge by our own services became a major challenge.

ESTABLISHING THE TEAM AND A STRATEGY

Establishing a team

In Autumn 1984, in an attempt to clarify the nature of the problem facing Camberwell, the Health Authority's Management Team decided to set up a group, convened by the Senior Planning Officer, to 'determine what would be the most appropriate alternative types of service provision for people from Camberwell who were currently patients at Cane Hill'. This was to include all the wards — acute, long-stay and elderly — and would be building on existing services in the District. The first step would be 'to draw up a survey methodology' designed to ascertain the characteristics of the patients and which wards they were on. It was chaired by a consultant who worked at Cane Hill and who also represented Camberwell at the Regional level and included two future members of the Resettlement Team (FH and AW). This group undertook several surveys and these were presented to the general management of the Maudsley and Camberwell Hospitals. The outcome was that a joint working group was convened in 1987 to steer the service development process, and a residential group was also established to examine options for future accommodation for the Cane Hill residents.

The steering group had senior representatives from Lambeth and Southwark, Camberwell Health Authority, Bethlem and Maudsley Health Authority, Housing Associations, the local National Schizophrenia Fellowship, and the CRT as they came into post. It continued meeting until 1989, when its functions were replaced by another similar group, and provided the direction and seniority to ensure that inevitable problems in the process of the developing new services could be smoothed over wherever possible.

The survey group meetings laid the basis for the policy of recruiting a multidisciplinary resettlement team.

Obstacles to establishing a team

The establishment of the team was not without difficulties. At this early stage (mid-1986) there was no financial support available and staff were redeployed from existing work within Camberwell's long-term mental illness service. In the words of one of the strongest advocates for the team, the Chairman of the Division of Psychiatry at King's:

> *'I am writing on behalf of my colleagues to express our grave concern about a number of issues relating to this task [the management of the 'running-down' of Cane Hill]. As you may know, Dr Tony Wainwright, Clinical Psychologist, Sue Wibley, Sister at the Psychiatric Day Hospital, and I have started work at Cane Hill Hospital to assess the needs of the long-stay patients... This work is being undertaken prior to the establishment of the Rehabilitation and Continuing Care team. It has meant that our existing clinical commitments have had to be reduced and we are seeking funding for locum cover, from the Community Unit General Manager.*

> *(May 1986)*

Furthermore the bid made for joint funding from Lambeth and Camberwell for the team was turned down. The initial reaction to the proposal for the team by the South East Thames Regional Health Authority was lukewarm mainly, so far as we could tell, on financial grounds but also because there was dispute about whether the costs should fall exclusively on Districts, Region, Local Authorities or what. As shown by the following lively response, we did not take it lying down.

> *'I write to express our dismay and anger as consultants in Psychiatry at King's on learning that our proposal for this team has not received financial support from South East Thames Regional Health Authority. I wish to say (speaking for all of us in the strongest terms) that this response from Region is totally unacceptable to us at King's.'*

> *(July 1986)*

The final agreement to fund the team came in late 1986, and the team was fully up to strength by March 1987.

Responsibilities of the team

Two interlinked areas were seen as high priority. First, to take on clinical responsibility for the 117 Cane Hill patients who had been admitted with 'functional mental illness' and to get to know them as well as possible so that, second, the planning of the replacement services would be closely informed by this knowledge. In the words of the Operational Policy (1988) we had 'to develop services that would replace those currently provided by Cane Hill Hospital for the functionally mentally ill long-term residents from Camberwell Health District' and 'to extend the community-based services for the long-term mentally ill who lived in the East Lambeth sector.'

The full scale of the work that was undertaken is shown in Figure 1.3. In this intervening period a small group (a nurse, a psychologist and a general manager) attempted to carry out some of the groundwork to allow the team to operate more effectively. A survey of local housing stock indicated what might be available at the expected affordable cost. On guesses on the sorts of problems the Cane Hill residents had, based on the surveys and face-to-face meetings, numbers of houses, staffing levels and support systems were made. An outline operational policy for the team was drawn up, including the principles they would work towards. This approach was substantially influenced by the ideas of this small team who had strong sympathies with Social Role Valorization (Wolfensberger, 1983). The emphasis would be on setting-up services where people would have the opportunity to lead as valued lives as possible. The process would be carried out in such a way that the individuals' wishes would be taken into account, and that they would be treated as citizens with the rights concomitant with that status.

A 'progress report' written in December 1986 indicated how far the plan for the future service had progressed before the full team came into post. The areas covered can usefully be summarized as follows:

1. A placement officer had been recruited and had begun to explore the private and voluntary sector. That this had such an early high profile shows the key role in the strategy it was seen as playing. Provided the services were up to standard, it was seen as a way of transferring costs from the National Health Service budget to that of the Department of Social Security. We were prepared to do deals with providers so that they could get higher rates than DHSS by 'topping up'. This was subsequently stopped by a decision taken by the Department of Health and communicated to Districts by the Chief Executive of the Health Service. The obvious problems here was that there was high pressure to move people to private accommodation, and less pressure to ensure that the quality was up to standard. We tried to set up methods to monitor this aspect by follow-up and evaluation.
2. Meetings had been held with housing associations with the aim of their providing the development work for housing. We were proposing single person flats and two-person flats in ordinary housing stock and a 12-place hostel. All ground floor flats were to be of mobility standard.
3. The method recommended by the Housing Association for running this accommodation was to be a 'Consortium', which would provide the service, but where the Health Authority would employ the staff. It would have the advantage of distancing the Health Authority from the finance of the housing so we could claim the DHSS Board and Lodging Allowance. It would also provide a forum that might help the different agencies involved to collaborate. The way the service was actually financed is shown in Figure 1.4.

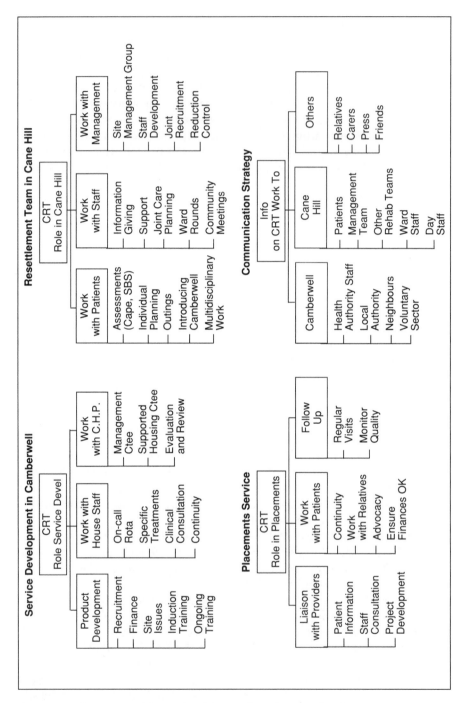

Figure 1.3   Summary of the scale of the work undertaken by the team.

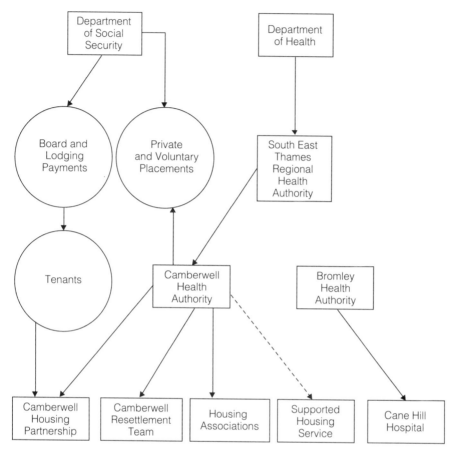

Figure 1.4 How the re-housing service was actually financed.

4. Meetings were held with the Director of Manpower Planning at King's College Hospital to agree the staffing for the housing service. At this time, estimates of the number required varied between 171 and 70 and large amounts of the nurse's and general manager's time were taken up in working out what was necessary.

Characteristics of the team

A question raised by the appointment of the team was the comparison of the skills mix chosen with tasks it had been called upon to perform. The tasks involved skills more usually associated with accountants, solicitors, housing workers, estate agents and so on. The team had therefore to develop these skills as it was essential that those planning the service had a good knowledge of the people for whom the planning was being done.

Planning can often be an empty exercise (Peck, 1985) and we wanted to avoid this. Nevertheless, it stretched the skills of the team and we had to learn an enormous amount as we went along. In general, the clinical tasks were well within the competence of the team. The service development tasks were much more learning by doing. The reasons for the establishment of this type of team were varied but two particular reasons stand out.

1. That multidisciplinary teams are what is needed in health services has become axiomatic. It is accepted uncritically on the whole, and since the staff proposing the team in this case were themselves hoping to become part of it, there were pressures to go for such a model, so that our work as individuals could continue.
2. The task was going to be highly political and necessarily would need senior staff who carried some clout in the organization. We had seen other teams set up without a consultant, for example, and these had been obstructed by others in the organization with differing priorities, and were eventually wound up. The high profile of the team was a conscious effort to ensure that the job got done, despite anticipated opposition.

The composition of the team from March 1987 was: (a) a placement officer; (b) a consultant psychiatrist; (c) a principal psychologist; (d) a senior nurse; (e) a clinical nurse specialist; and (f) a locum occupational therapist. In addition, joint finance was obtained for a full-time Lambeth social worker, and a Southwark social worker who had been associated with Cane Hill Hospital for many years joined us. Subsequent recruitment included two further nurses for the team, two nurses for the placement service and a part-time occupational therapist.

Summary of team strengths and weaknesses

One team member summarized his view of the team's strengths and weaknesses in a recent presentation (Holloway, 1990; Fig. 1.5).

Undertaking too many roles. As can be seen from Figure 1.3 the span of operations of the team's work was very wide. The team members also wished to actively pursue all these areas as they offered varied and interesting experiences. It was an exciting time, and our skills increased. Another aspect of this issue was the tendency of members of the team to be lured away to support other aspects of the Camberwell services. The senior nurse became involved in the acute unit and eventually was providing very little input to the resettlement process and the psychologist took over providing supervision for the other nurses. The consultant had responsibilities for 'community psychiatry' in Camberwell (such things as the Day Hospital), and this ate into his time. I took on the role of Acting District Psychologist in January 1989 and this took me away from the team. This set

- Undertaking too many roles
- Inexperienced in the workings of a large psychiatric hospital
- Inexperienced in traditional psychiatric rehabilitation
- Inexperienced in planning on the scale required
- Lack of experience in community-based residential services
- Distrust of assessment techniques and unable to implement care planning
- Initial ideological disagreements
- Blurred authority and accountability
- Possessive about our patients
- Committed to client group
- Effective multidisciplinary working
- Applied a range of personal and professional skills to the task
- No longer inexperienced!

Figure 1.5 Skills and weaknesses of the Camberwell resettlement team (after Holloway, 1990).

up considerable tensions and for some time there were two teams in operation with somewhat overlapping membership. One was working primarily with the patients at Cane Hill, and was referred to as the clinical team, and the other worked mostly on service development.

Inexperience in the workings of a large psychiatric hospital and in traditional psychiatric rehabilitation. Although we had all been working in the area of long-term mental health, none of us were prepared for the complex politics of Cane Hill. We were shown up in this respect by comparison with the Lewisham and North Southwark team, which was led by Dr Isobel Morris, a clinical psychologist who had been closely involved in the setting up of the Maudsley services for this client group in the late 1970s. She had also been most recently working in Friern Hospital, which had a major closure programme under way. Her approach was instructive and very effective: her starting point was to value highly and genuinely the work that was being done in the hospital. By taking this approach, she was able to get the best out of the staff. In addition, she was able to read the needs of the organization and, at a crucial point in the process when the hospital was desperate to retain training status for nurses, she put in a proposal to have an integrated training ward for the Lewisham patients. The hospital management agreed and the Lewisham team had the lion's share of funds spent on their service.

In contrast, we were attending to the more gloomy aspects of the Cane Hill system and were often in conflict with the managers. Also, we were unable to see the extent to which our own future was bound up with that of the managers. Our lack of experience in traditional rehabilitation resulted in a clash of methods between our approach based on a more social approach and those practised at the hospital. It meant we again were not able initially to get the best out of the system.

Inexperience in planning on the scale required. There is no doubt that the team would have benefited from members who had planning experience on a relevant scale. The input from a planning officer from District was of great help in the early stages, as he had been a leading player in the closure of Darenth Park Hospital, and also in the subsequent development of the Camberwell service for people with learning difficulties. For the rest of us, the politics of planning were new. The fact that there was a planning cycle, for example, meant that bids had to be in Region by a date known in advance. As we were not aware of this to start with, we could not understand the pressure applied to us from time to time for information on proposed projects.

Lack of experience in community-based residential services. In setting up the supported houses we had models from other services to draw on; however, none of us had worked as, for example, a residential social worker. This would have been a distinct advantage in having some understanding of which patients could manage in which settings. Alternatively, it may have allowed us to avoid being prejudiced so that we tried things we otherwise might have avoided.

Distrust of assessment techniques and inability to implement care planning. Our methods for assessing people depended on spending time with them in as many situations as possible and using this experience to describe the person. I personally distrust an over-reliance on formal assessment methods if they are used to suggest where people should be placed (e.g. Clifton Assessment Procedure for the Elderly — CAPE) as they may be the vehicle for self-fulfilling prophecies. However, such scales were used as well as others; however, the conclusions drawn from them were never used in a way to strongly influence the patterns of care in the hospital. Our main method of influencing care was through discussions with the staff, and the occasional use of monitoring methods for things such as continence problems. The care planning issue may have arisen from our distance from the Cane Hill staff; as this distance has decreased, we have been increasingly successful. Care planning in the Supported Housing Service has not been well implemented, and that may also have derived from our lack of commitment to the process.

Initial ideological disagreements. From the outset there were ideological differences between team members . These centred on the definition of the problem: whether it was primarily a problem of mental illness and secondary handicaps, or of social disadvantage and devaluation. These issues have been discussed elsewhere in relation to the outcome of an evaluation of a Day Hospital in Camberwell (Wainwright *et al.*, 1988). Using an approach based on normalization, one set of conclusions were drawn; using a more traditional approach another set of conclusions emerged. The differences were not insurmountable and centred more on what should be given priority. Should the future residents be protected from society, or should social integration be our aim? Was imagery important or not? These issues are further explored in Wainwright and Lindley (1991). An illustration of how these divisions affected our practice is found in the way we decided to develop the 'high-support' house. From one perspective, this was regarded as a possible 'home for life' for the residents; from the other it was regarded as a rehabilitation facility, albeit long-term. These two positions would lead to rather different operational policies and different expectations of the residents. The view that it should be a rehabilitation facility gained ground, with the proviso that this service should be provided in as non-stigmatizing a way as possible. The discussions of the plans were heated and difficult but necessary.

Blurred authority and accountability. Leadership of the team was a difficult area that was partly alleviated by identifying different 'leadership functions' (Watts and Bennett, 1983). Different meetings were chaired by different members of the team in an attempt to spread these functions. While this led to some definite advantages, and has contributed to the strength of the team, it covered up a fundamental difference in status of team members. One member commented that 'the team includes a mix of grades and responsibilities which is unhelpful in facilitating efficient decision-making'. The consultant, the senior nurse manager and the psychologist, together with the general manager, formed the executive of the team, and met in several formal and informal guises. The avoidance of deciding which of these four people would be **the leader** became increasingly difficult as, both for internal and external reasons, an individual was needed as the co-ordinator. This issue at some stages may have been played out disguised as ideological differences. To avoid the conflict between the clinicians, the manager was given the task of team leader, although he never appeared to grasp the title, and perhaps six months to one year later was, due to the priority of the Cane Hill work slipping down the agenda, no longer part of the team. Subsequently, the consultant became team leader by common consent, as the threat to the existence of the team posed by integration with the Special Health Authority required a submerging of individual differences and the promotion of a strong image. Strong teams are led by consultants, at least they are in Camberwell.

Possessive attitude towards patients. The methods that were adopted involved developing strong personal commitments to the patients. While this allowed us to work with people who had little by way of consistent support, it meant that handing over the service to the Supported Housing staff was quite hard. This process is still in train.

Commitment to the client group. The core members of the team were committed to working with people with long-term mental ill-health as it was their area of expertise. The client group did not generally enjoy a high status and had been relatively neglected by professionals. As a team we enjoyed working in this area and regarded it as long overdue that the clients received a good service and a substantially improved quality of life. Nevertheless, there remained substantial differences between team members; these were primarily interpersonal rather than interdisciplinary. Therefore the agreed strategy was clearly a compromise. Although I did not feel a nursing home with 20 places for elderly people was a valued way to support them, I accepted this as there were no alternatives that could be agreed upon. In practice, a nursing home was not forthcoming and the service may be substantially worse off as a result. Favouring as I do the importance of social integration, I argued against congregating more than four or five people at the most in one place. Others argued that the residents would find that situation too intense and that ten to 15 was quite acceptable. They argued that even 20 was not a problem as social integration was not seen as being of particularly high priority, as it was superseded by day care, or high-quality nursing care.

Effective multidisciplinary team-working and applying a range of skills to the task. The members of the team provided complementary skills and were able to share their professional competence in a very effective way. This undoubtedly benefited the patients since they had input from several different specialists in addressing their problems (Gowler and Parry, 1979; Ovretveit, 1986). The team made a commitment to try and produce a synthesis between the different approaches, which, in practice, was possible as the common concerns of basic good practice were shared and were embodied in the 'Coming Home to Camberwell' strategy (Wainwright, 1987).

Increased experience. It is something of a truism that the team is now in a much better position to understand the nature of the task of hospital closure just as it is ending. (It has been suggested that perhaps we should hire ourselves out as hospital closure consultants.) The team had also to change its style as it had to face different challenges as the service developed. At the start there was the issue of working in an existing institution, coupled with raising awareness in Camberwell. Later, as the new services came 'on-line', the team had to progressively give up responsibilities, which was a difficult process at times.

General summary

The Operational policy of the team was completed in 1987 after the remaining members had been recruited. It explicitly omitted the term 'normalization' from its philosophy, but attempted to incorporate the notions from Social Role Valorization as well as a Community Psychiatry approach.

(Community Psychiatry regards 'the problem' faced by services as principally located in the individual, their symptoms, antisocial behaviour and the like, and that the most effective setting in which to treat such patients is in the community. Social Role Valorization regards 'the problem' as being principally located in a society's response to differences that are negatively valued.) This approach was taken because normalization had been the ideological framework that had guided the development of the local learning difficulties service and this service was in some turmoil and normalization was being blamed for its problems. Furthermore, the team's own internal debates on the rights and wrongs of the approach needed to be contained. The primary aim of the team was therefore stated as:

> *'...the reduction of the disabilities experienced by the mentally ill. Disabilities include the specific psychological or biological impairments occurring during an episode of illness.'*

It also committed itself to the notion that:

> *'People who have long-term mental illnesses have the same rights as other citizens. Those providing the service will promote personal choice and protect individual rights. In order for the users' own wishes to be taken into account, mechanisms should be provided within the service and are specified in the 'code of practice'.*

> *(Operational Policy, March 1987)*

How far these principles were adhered to has been a major concern for the team and remains an area of debate. Within the team, whether people will be suitable for one placement or another is carefully discussed **prior** to discussing it with the persons involved. It is very rare for people to be a party to these debates — so much for being treated with the same rights as other citizens. Furthermore, in the supported housing service, the concern to regard the tenant as an individual may over-ride the need to develop intensive systematic programmes of support. On one occasion, when discussing a person who presented many challenges to the service, I asked the team whether they had considered developing a consistent approach to the person. They replied that they did not feel that was appropriate as they all had their own individual relationships with the person and it would interfere with them.

The team's strategy to develop services to replace Cane Hill Hospital

The development of a 'robust' (financially viable) strategy for the new services was a high priority for the Camberwell managers. Much money was at stake and, in the context of regular overspending by the District and Government demands for efficiency savings, the closure of Cane Hill was seen as a potential 'pot of gold'. By May 1988, an option appraisal had been drawn up by the Resettlement Team based on a strategic plan for the District, which was approved in 1987. An estimated provisional income for Cane Hill and related services was over £3 million per year, of which over £2 million went straight to Bromley Health Authority to run Cane Hill. The sooner the patients could be got out, the sooner the money would be available locally.

Major financial problems faced Camberwell with the change in Regional funding policy, which took place in March 1988. Prior to this date the Region had undertaken to indemnify the District against the inevitable rise in unit costs that occurs when a hospital reduces the number of patients. To explain this, one only has to consider the case of a single ward with 20 patients. If ten are discharged to a project, the running costs of the ward remain substantially the same, as it has to be heated and staffed in much the same way as before, thus the cost per patient will double. In addition, costs rise faster than inflation.

After March 1988, the Districts were compelled to contract with Bromley Health Authority on behalf of Cane Hill for a definite number of beds each quarter in advance. These changes had the effect of substantially increasing the costs of providing care for patients at Cane Hill, estimated at that time as approximately an extra £250 000 over three years. However, the shortfall did not materialize and, in February 1989, the Region agreed to transitional funding in 1989/90 of £400 000, and in 1990/91 of £500 000. The fact that we could not predict this in 1988 illustrates that throughout the process uncertainty in funding determined planning decisions, which in a more stable climate might have been different.

While the option appraisal paper was being written, a strategy that would go to the Health Authority as the basis for our work over the next five years was being constructed. We worked hard on this document and had a draft to the relevant managers within six months of the team coming into post. It was called 'Coming Home to Camberwell'. As less than one third will in fact do so, the title in retrospect is somewhat ironic. It was with some frustration that the team watched while financial wrangling prevented the publication of the strategy until approximately one year later. The main elements of the strategy are outlined in Figures 1.6 and 1.7.

The strategy was produced as a guide to our own activities, but also as a way of informing the local authorities, voluntary organizations and staff, both at Cane Hill and locally, of our intentions. Importantly, it also allowed us to state what was necessary as a minimum, and that shortcomings of the final service could be assessed against it (compare with Figure 1.8, which outlines the services that have been developed). The numbers we were planning for depended on estimates of 'attrition', the rather ugly fact that many people would die over our five-year planning period. The average death rate in the hospital had been about 10% per year, which may seem high but many of the residents were very elderly, and the people with dementia in particular had a short life-expectancy after admission. Given this figure one might expect the 117 people who were in our group at the

- CONSUMER ORIENTATED
  promote and safeguard personal rights
  maintain and enhance dignity
  take carers views into account
  take carers needs into account
  avoid stigmatising service images
  encourage integration with non-handicapped
  incorporate a clients charter of rights

- EQUAL OPPORTUNITIES
  non-discriminatory
  promote the interests of the handicapped

- INTEGRATED
  multi-agency and multi-disciplinary

- FLEXIBLE
  to meet changing needs of clients/service

- COMMUNITY BASED
  people to live in 'ordinary housing'

- OPEN
  to external and internal audit
  effective quality assurance in place

Figure 1.6   Service principles reflected in the strategy of the Camberwell team.

- **Clients**
  32 East Lambeth
  27 South Southwark
  27 stateless
  Average length of stay 25 years
  Average age 66 years
  26 aged less than 60 years

- **Accommodation planned**
  28 places in staffed housing
  12 places in rehabilitation hostel
  20 places in elderly nursing home
   4 places in cluster flats
   8 places for 'challenging bahaviour'
  14 private placements or less depending on when people die

- **Other planned services**
  Cafe cum social club
  Resource centre/office base
  Sheltered work
  Citizen advocacy service
  Social and recreation budget

- **Other services**
  Continuing access to the resettlement team
  Equal access to general medical services

Figure 1.7   The 'Coming Home to Camberwell' strategy.

```
■ Accommodation provided
  20 places in staffed housing
  10 places in rehabilitation hostel
   0 places in elderly nursing home
   0 places in cluster flats
   ? places for 'challenging behaviour'
  Over 30 private placements

■ Other planned services
  The 48 club
  Southside Rehabilitation Association
  Lambeth Forum/Lambeth Link
  Social and recreation budget

■ Other services
  Continuing access to the resettlement team
  Equal acccess to general medical services
```

Figure 1.8   Outcome of closure of the Cane Hill Hospital.

start to have dropped to about 69 by 1991, and indeed that was the case. As you can imagine all the members of the team attended a few funerals during this work, and this may be partly seen as a price to be paid for the style of support the team offered. This emphasized, however, that the number of replacement places in the strategy would only cover the remaining patients, and would not be able to fund large service developments for people becoming unwell in the District.

The implementation of the strategy

The four houses were opened in 1989 and provided 21 places. One place has since been lost due to registration requirements. The hostel is projected to open in November 1991. The Social Club is open and is managed by the Mental After Care Association. The work programme is on track to open later this year managed by a charity, the Southside Rehabilitation Association, set up by the team. The advocacy service in the form of Lambeth Link has been rapidly expanding over the past 18 months and is now a very effective consumer organization.

The strategy lost some elements. The two major losses were the nursing home and the resource centre. The former was dropped because of capital funding difficulties at regional level, and lack of available building space in the District at an affordable price. The consequence of this is a local shortfall of places for elderly people needing this type of support. The resource centre was simply not funded, and we were faced with a choice of either the hostel or the centre. The Region's capital problems were a reflection of the economic climate at the time and poor estimates of available funds from land sales. The other change was due to a scaling down of the numbers of people the team felt would be able to be supported in the staffed accommodation that we were providing and a lack of agreement on imaginative community-based solutions for people with challenging behaviour.

The use of private placements was the service area that expanded substantially, the numbers placed being over twice as many as originally envisaged. It is easy to see in retrospect that there were such strong forces moving us in that direction that it was somewhat inevitable. Particularly in the early stages of the process when we were learning as we went along, we took each placement very seriously since we were deciding on the future life of the people being placed. (The essentials of the service are described in Booker *et al.*, 1989.) Moving house is a very emotional process for everyone, and for people who have lived somewhere for decades it is almost inevitably a tremendous wrench. The team members shared in these feelings as we had relationships with the patients, which made it matter to us that things went well for them.

The model chosen for the new housing service was to set up a consortium (defined as a 'temporary co-operation of large interests to effect some common purpose') to manage the houses. The 'large interests' were Camberwell and the Bethlem/Maudsley Health Authorities, Lambeth and Southwark, Housing Associations, and voluntary sector groups. It was envisaged that this would provide a forum for interested parties and, in addition, permit the charging of board and lodging payments, thus shifting some of the costs on to the Social Security budget. The emphasis on multi-agency involvement was important, but very difficult to achieve in practice. The Camberwell Housing Partnership was set up in summer of 1988, at which time its director was employed. It was originally envisaged that this organization would manage all the successor services; however, it has had some major problems and, in April 1991, merged with a similar consortium for people with learning difficulties to form a larger 'social care agency'. The structure had built-in problems of authority with staff employed by the Health Authority, the houses owned by the housing associations, and the Partnership responsible for the service.

The management committee had responsibility without authority and did not function well. It was drawn from professional staff involved in the development of the houses. There was severe role confusion. One example was that the Chairperson was the consultant on the resettlement team, and I am the Chair of the supported housing subcommittee. There was a major loss of financial control and direction, which could be attributed to the poor function of the management committee and the performance of the development worker in the main. It has been a lesson to learn from. Managing a voluntary organization is a major responsibility that cannot be performed in someone's spare time unless there is a very effective officer team.

The impact of the complex service system

There have been major changes in the way the NHS is managed during the past five years. The introduction of the Griffiths reforms brought Sainsbury's style General Management and the NHS and Community Care Act 1990 has brought contracts and NHS trusts. In addition, our two local authorities have been in a state of continual reorganization as well as being 'rate-/charge-capped'. These issues may be common to many other places, especially deprived inner-city services like ours. However, the additional problem we faced was the move towards the Bethlem/Maudsley group managing Camberwell's mental health services. The issues are too complex and too parochial to describe here, but it would be hard to underestimate the amount of time the issue took up.

The two authorities had been toying with the notion for many years. Rivalry kept them apart but finally, in 1984, the Hospital Advisory Service recommended a merger, and since then they have been painfully inching into each other's arms. To illustrate the problems, final integration was to take place on April 1st (appropriately enough) 1991, and a week before it was due to happen (or not!) the two sides could not agree about the 'financial package', which may have had to involve the Minister. The impact of all this on our planning was considerable. We attempted to involve them in our meetings, and sometimes we managed it, sometimes we did not. There was generally an air of hostility to our proposals since they felt that **they** should have the Cane Hill money and not us, although how we were to plan the service was never very clear. On our side, we wrote the strategy without mentioning the way that the Bethlem/Maudsley services would be involved, simply noting that they would be and that:

> '...the service plan...has been designed in such a way as to be compatible with such a change in management arrangements...'.

This was because we were unable to gain any clear picture from them or our own management team of how the integration would affect us. Members of the Bethlem/Maudsley service criticized us for this, viewing our plans as a 'bolt-on approach' rather than being integrated with their existing services. We are hoping that after integration this area will improve.

Quite apart from our own local complexities, Cane Hill was very complex in its own right. In brief, it was owned by the South East Thames Region, managed by Bromley Health Authority and physically located in Croydon Health Authority. The other interested Health Authorities that had patients there were Camberwell, Bethlem and Maudsley, Lewisham and North Southwark and West Lambeth. The Local Authorities involved were Bromley, Lambeth, Southwark, Lewisham, Croydon. All these agencies at one time or another had important issues concerning the closure of the hospital, which presented the Bromley management with a very major challenge. For our resettlement team, it was important to keep our own plans in line with others and this took up much time, particularly in the first eighteen months.

HOSPITAL TO HOUSES AND PRIVATE PLACEMENTS

The patient group

When we started at the hospital, our information was largely contained in a survey carried out in January 1986, which gave us a broad view of the patients. Their average age was 66 years, with 15% under 50 and 71% over 60. Over 80% had a diagnosis of psychosis. The average length of stay was 23 years, with 13% less than five years and 34% more than 30 years. The number of compulsory patients was 5%. Only 7% had spent some time out of hospital during their admission.

In terms of the estimated level of performance that the patients were functioning at, 24% were considered to be high to moderate, 48% low to very poor. The latter were considered to require 24-hour care. In terms of physical health, nearly 70% were in reasonable health, although about a quarter suffered from incontinence. The survey reported low levels of social contacts, although about a third participated in some sort of programmed activity in the hospital. Less than half (44%) were thought to have behavioural problems severe enough to affect residential placement. A third of the patients were identified as 'hard to place' with a variety of problems requiring a variety of particular solutions (Clifford, 1986). This information was useful as a guide but it was recognized that it was no substitute for getting to know the individuals and carrying out the process of individual assessment, which would be the team's initial task.

Relationships with the hospital staff

When we started working at the hospital, the management consisted of a 'Site Management Group' (SMG) chaired by the Director of Nursing Services. It was during the first year of our work that general management was introduced. This faced the internal managers with a joint challenge. On the one hand, there were the resettlement teams and their respective Districts organizing to pull out all their resources and, on the other, the Bromley General Managers who wanted to pull resources out of the hospital for their own developments. This set up considerable strains, which we could only witness from a distance. It posed problems for us because our perception was that they became, not unreasonably, rather suspicious and we therefore found it difficult to gain close access to their deliberations. Our lack of experience in the way mental hospitals ran compounded this and, in the words of the consultant on our team, we were 'had for breakfast, several times'. Suffice it to say, relations were strained for some time. One early event did not help. Following a letter written by one of the Camberwell hospital managers, who happened also to be project worker for Lambeth MIND, there had been a major explosion of feeling against the Camberwell team. He had visited the hospital in 1986 with a member of the team and wrote the following statement, copying it to the Community Health Councils in Camberwell and Bromley.

'I am writing to express my feelings of disgust whilst in Cane Hill last week. I passed through...ward on 10th June in order to visit a member of the Camberwell Community team who was interviewing patients on the ward. As you may be aware, people admitted to this ward are most frequently from the Camberwell area. Discharges from this ward are mainly due to the death of the patient, a fact which I am sure will not have escaped their attention. However, far from the staff developing the skills required to deal with this issue during their interactions with patients, the staff on [ ] appear to have developed a more confrontational approach which I find totally unacceptable.'

He noted that the 'last offices box' (used when 'laying-out' a deceased person) was in full view of the patients, and that a sign had been 'sello-taped' to the door of the locker from Bromley crematorium giving details of a patient's death and the various prices for headstones and the like.

The outcome of this was that the staff were very suspicious of Camberwell for some time after and this became known as 'the Camberwell syndrome' in which the team was considered to have behaved badly and betrayed a trust.

The person who became the General Manager of the hospital was the finance officer for the Mental Health Unit and a member of the SMG. He was very successful in getting the finances of the organization under control and, very quickly, was able to make good relationships with the resettlement teams. As time went on, however, retrenchment of hospital facilities and the needs of the resettlement team came into conflict more and more.

The reduction control plan

In order to co-ordinate the retrenchment of the hospital with the plans of each District, the Hospital Manager convened a meeting to support him in writing the Reduction Control Plan document, a strategy for closing the hospital in an orderly manner. The team members played an important role here, attending meetings with information about projects as they became finalized, about details of slippage and related matters. The meetings were also to co-ordinate ward closures, which would result in patients being moved. Before the arrival of the teams such closures would happen with little warning for either staff or patients. On one occasion, even after we had started, the team consultant arrived at the hospital for a ward round, only to find the ward had closed and his patients had been moved elsewhere within the hospital.

We devised a plan for a Camberwell sector within the hospital. This would have had a single manager, and would contain all the Camberwell patients. The notion was that we could then co-ordinate our work across the small number of wards more effectively and relate to the hospital better. We felt that we may have been able to recruit Camberwell nursing staff to work in the unit, who would then move out with the patients. This was rejected by the management as unworkable. I feel now that if we had a better understanding of mental hospital politics we could have seen that it would have been turned down sooner and gone for the Lewisham model of upgrading a single ward as a teaching unit, as that gave the hospital something, and was not perceived as for the benefit of the resettlement team alone. The hospital had a potent rumour mill, many connected with the idea that closure of the hospital was to be much faster than planned, because of shortage of staff and other considerations. The Reduction Control Plan meeting was a useful forum for checking some of these, and it played a useful role in the closure programme.

Staff development

The Camberwell team played a significant role in organizing and establishing a staff development group for the Bromley staff. We held a series of workshops for senior managers; these were taken over subsequently by the Regional Training Team, the Bromley team and the School of Nursing, which have developed an English National Board approved course. The nursing middle management have a development programme supported by the region. In general, there was a poor personnel policy with no collaboration between the three districts. In 1987, I made several attempts to bring the personnel departments together, but eventually gave up. When staff wanted to know if they would be able to work in Camberwell services they could only be given vague answers. This area is a major one in terms of managing the process. In other closure programmes very generous personnel policies were in place and made the whole process much more tolerable for the staff (c.f. the Exeter experience; see King, 1988).

Relations with nurses

Despite the upset over the personnel policy, we had made it a central objective to get to know the staff well, and the nurses on the team played the central role in this task. The Camberwell patients were scattered over 11 wards. There were two that were designated for Camberwell patients — the rest had a mixture of people from different districts. All the nursing staff were Bromley employees and the majority of management staff had worked there for many years, the Director of Nursing Services starting in 1968. Our nurses, being Camberwell staff, had no authority over Bromley nurses, even if more junior than them. Also, because the Bromley staff had extremely limited information about the future, were threatened by our presence and were low in morale, during the first six months much effort was put into spending time in the wards and on the units answering questions about our programme and the work we were doing in the hospital and elsewhere. This was because good working relationships with the nurses were crucial. The staffing levels in the hospital were poor and, on occasion, there would be a nursing auxiliary in charge of a ward of 30 people. This made the task even harder as there was often little continuity across wards and, on occasion, the standard of nursing care was not very good. In a note I took at the time I wrote that:

> 'The most striking aspect of the current provision for our patients is the extremely poor level of staff input. This applies across the disciplines and represents a serious obstacle to any realistic programme of rehabilitation. Nursing cover varies from very limited to seriously inadequate. An additional source of concern is food provided for the patients. There have been reports from other hospitals, particularly those catering for the elderly, of malnutrition. The impression we have is that patients are at risk of suffering in this way... Personal respect for such things as death seems to be slipping. On one ward it was only the intervention of a nurse already involved in another medical problem who saved the patients being exposed to two porters loading a corpse on to a trolley and wheeling it out in full view.'

> *(Wainwright, 1987)*

However intermittent these issues were, they set the tone for our feelings about the hospital and influenced our work. The nurses on the team took the title of Camberwell Liaison Nurses and divided their energy between the different areas.

Relations with medical staff

The medical staff were mainly Bromley Health Authority employees, although there was one Lewisham and North Southwark Consultant and there were two Camberwell consultants. All the long-stay patients were the clinical responsibility of Bromley consultants until the Consultant member of the resettlement team, an Honorary Consultant with Bromley, took over. He continued to have junior doctor support from Bromley. On the whole, relations were not problematic. The Camberwell team consultant was able to mediate any difficulties that arose, and for most of the time there was no need for active collaboration.

Relations with other departments

The Occupational Therapy Department on the whole linked in well with the Resettlement Team, although there were in fact only two qualified occupational therapists (OTs) for a relatively large department, which consisted of occupational therapy helpers who had worked in the hospital for some time and were very experienced. The OT on the Resettlement Team (when we had one) liaised well with this department. Occasionally, there were difficulties in getting access to occupational therapy facilities and there was some suspicion that Bromley were at times getting a rather better deal. The Social and Recreational staff were in many ways the most energetic and enthusiastic and were headed up by a nurse, who had changed his duties during the course of his work at Cane Hill over many years, to become the Head of the Social and Recreational Service. He started up the 'Pop-in', an on-site cafe, which generated its own income to provide extra activities for the patients. The working relationship with this service has been very valuable.

In contrast, our relationship with the secretarial system has always been rather strained and it was never clear whether the Resettlement Team had real access to a secretarial service or not. The consultant was able to have a fairly reasonable secretarial service and, from time to time, other members of the Team used the secretarial time at the hospital but it was generally regarded as not very available. The secretarial service includes members who have worked at the hospital for a substantial period of time and are quite influential and have, at times, affected clinical decision-making.

The Bromley Social Work Department at Cane Hill have a small staff, again, who were experienced and knew the patients well. When we first arrived in 1986, we were met with some ambivalence, both welcomed and rejected simultaneously. Lambeth did not provide social work support for the patients at Cane Hill, despite patients being admitted from Lambeth. This is, in fact, normal practice for out-of-area hospitals. Nevertheless it resulted in sufficiently strong feelings for one social worker to say to us on our arrival about the Lambeth Social Work Department that 'they bring their shit and dump it on our doorstep and refuse to take it away!' However, in time excellent working relationships between the Social Work Department and the Lambeth social worker on our team grew up.

Relating to the other resettlement teams

In 1984, the Bromley team was set up as a nursing team who were to be supernumerary to the ward staff but increasingly were absorbed into carrying out ward duties to cover sickness and so on. This team was dissolved in 1986 and reconstituted in 1987 as a full team and they, together with the Lewisham and North Southwark team, shared a ward with the Camberwell team. While the three teams shared a single ward, we had meetings to compare the ways in which we were developing strategies, and reading groups and seminars were similarly held. However, this was rather intermittent and the cross-talk between the teams was largely informal. There was also some competition between the teams because resources were at a premium.

The teams each had a different relationship with the hospital management. For the Bromley team, they were both part of and not part of the Bromley service, being seen as coming in from outside and yet being part of Bromley Mental Health Unit. The Lewisham team had a Consultant who had clinical responsibility for their long-term patients as part of their team and his influence, together with the experience of the Principal Psychologist and the strategy they laid out for the way the work was to be organized, allowed them to work with the hospital staff and the hospital managers more effectively than the other two teams. Camberwell had been there for the longest but had considerable difficulty in overcoming some of the suspicion that the Bromley staff felt: (a) for a team coming in from outside; and (b) the historical antagonism felt towards the Maudsley and King's Hospitals. At times, information was probably not shared between the teams, so that one team could gain an advantage over another.

Individual 'assessment'

Team members were faced with a dual task that was firstly to develop a positive relationship with each person (patient), and secondly to have an informed opinion about the most appropriate way to support the person in the future, when they left hospital.

There are no formal or informal assessment methods that allow accurate prediction on a person's ability to do well in any particular community setting and this steered us away from any over-elaborate assessment methods. Although not used systematically, the ideas of Brost and Johnson (1982) were influential to us; these contain the notion of 'getting to know a person' rather than simply 'assessing a patient'. We collected information on each person by informal methods, which included spending time with them in different settings and observing their abilities, talking with the person, talking with staff and others who knew them. In addition, more formal methods were used; these involved the Social Performance Schedule, behaviour monitoring charts, and checklists. Mental state examinations were regularly carried out by the medical staff. The 'assessment' work fell largely to the nurses and social workers, although we all contributed in different ways with different individuals.

The patients were hard to convince that anything was really going to happen. They had seen the number of people living with them in the hospital steadily decreasing and yet the hospital was still there, embodying a permanence and unshakable strength. We put out leaflets, talked to people, showed videos of Camberwell and got local papers delivered to the wards. This was a time of confidence building and paying particular attention to the emotional aspects of the patients' situation. We instituted community meetings on the two Camberwell wards — a novelty in the hospital. During this time we were given some 'pithy' feedback on our plans. One man who I asked about the hospitals closing said that we had put him in there for his nervous debility that was no better now than when he came in, so why were we asking him to leave? The community meetings raised many questions about practical things like money, who would do their cooking, where would they get clothes from and so on. It was a time of considerable anxiety as it sank in that the hospital really was closing and they would all have to leave:

> *More recent community meetings have taken on a distinctly more political edge, such as a ward community meeting with the group of patients who will be among the last to leave. The staff and patients are considering the food available and its lack of variety. The catering manager has been invited and is explaining that each patient is allocated £1.14 per day and so it is not surprising that the food is pretty poor. The resettlement team is there in force and continues to identify with the patients and remains outraged by the conditions in the hospital. The consultant points out that the average person spends 20% of their budget on food, while the patients are allocated 1% as it costs about £40 000 a year to keep them in Cane Hill Hospital. The patients are encouraged to write to the Community Health Council and the hospital authorities.*

The outcome was that the food improved and the communication with the caterers got better, but the charge nurse was ticked off for stepping out of line!

We took a decision to spend relatively little time in developing active rehabilitation programmes as many of the patients had gone through such programmes and had relapsed. We were dealing with people who had often been regarded as failures in placement terms. In addition, despite many hours spent in trying to get them, there were no rehabilitation facilities on the wards and so the scope for such programmes was limited. Some team members also realized that there was little purpose in teaching someone to cook in a situation where they did not have to cook, and could not cater for themselves even if they had wanted to mainly because of hospital rules. This work would be postponed to when they moved into the houses.

The emphasis was therefore on trying to form a strong relationship with the patients and thus learn how best to support them when they moved to their new homes. We went shopping with them to the local village, and on outings to Camberwell to shows and other social events. A trip to Camberwell in a car to see a house would have been a totally new experience, as they had not travelled that far in a car for many years. We learned quickly that people who have not had the experience get car sick a lot! Some groups were also run, for example a women's group. This was felt to be important as the hospital is a very 'male' environment and it is hard for women to maintain a strong identity. Another was a lunch group, which catered for four people at a time for a six-week period. This group gleaned such things as the fact that many people were reluctant to serve others with food and sharing tasks was very hard for some people.

Information was collected in this way and there was clearly a large measure of overlap between assessment and preparation for the move. A survey carried out in 1988 (Thorneycroft, 1988) showed that 75% of the patients did not know that the hospital was closing. Out of all the patients, 16% wanted to leave, 55% wanted to stay in the hospital now, 35% wanted to stay indefinitely and less than half the patients found the treatment they were receiving helpful.

Relatives' opinions were also mixed, and generally somewhat hostile. In fact few people had active contact with relatives, around three quarters never having visitors, and regrettably the way the relatives were informed led to considerable confusion and distress. In most cases, we were unable to tell the relatives anything definite about the future for their relative, apart from the fact that it would not be in Cane Hill, and would probably be in Camberwell. We could not even tell them with any degree of accuracy when their relatives would be likely to be moving. This initial confusion alerted us to the importance of being extremely careful of relatives' feelings and wishes, so members of the team put much effort into keeping them informed as things progressed. This has not prevented mistakes however. One recently occurred when we placed someone in a nursing home and the relative had been kept up-to-date with the plans. Shortly after the person had moved out, I had an understandably very concerned relative on the phone asking why they had received a bill for over £2300! Fortunately it was a mistake, but it may well have damaged future working relationships as apologies do not really undo the pain that such things inflict.

Rehabilitation in the hospital

Our main resource for rehabilitation was the upgraded Industrial Therapy Unit known as the John Hutchinson Centre, which was named after a well-remembered Cane Hill consultant. It had been losing clients steadily, and was unsustainable in the form in which it had been traditionally operating. Our team played an active role in planning the rehabilitation unit that replaced it and the Camberwell patients had a good deal of use out of it. The unit had a purpose-built kitchen so that it was possible for the groups to be held there. There was also a washing machine, and some patients opted to do their own washing so they could keep more control over their clothing.

Setting up the first houses

Although we have opened four houses, this account will concentrate on the first house as a case example. The Camberwell Housing Partnership which was to manage the service was being set up and finally was incorporated in June 1988. A development officer was appointed soon after. It is worth noting that this was not a clever way to have organized things, as too many decisions were needed before his appointment, and this order of things contributed much to the later problems of poor communication and collaboration between the team and the development officer.

House purchase and the project team

The first house was purchased in early 1987 and a project team to oversee its development was initiated in May of that year. The membership of this project team was mainly drawn from the resettlement team. It was hoped that it would come 'on-line' in September 1988, which provided the long lead time that we felt we needed as we were still learning as we went along. In fact, it slipped badly and finally opened in the same month as the second house in July 1989. We had also hoped to have a good gap between the opening of the other houses, but this did not really happen either as the third house opened in September 1989. The fourth house was opened in January 1990.

The project team decided that the first house would be for men for four main reasons. Firstly, none of the potential tenants for the houses lived in mixed facilities in the hospital and thus they had no recent experience of shared living with the opposite sex. Secondly, there were more men than women among the patients. Thirdly, the women in particular were not keen to share with men at that stage. Fourthly, the women were relatively more disabled, and there were a group of men who seemed keen to move and were likely to be better able to cope.

Design

All the houses were terraced, ordinary houses in ordinary streets. The internal design was to be as typical of an ordinary dwelling as possible. Fire regulations made this somewhat difficult at times as we had to have extinguishers, and fire alarms. In addition, the need to have lobbies to prevent fire spreading meant that some precious communal space was lost.

Selecting the residents

Selecting the people who would be offered a place in the project was done by a mixture of logical consideration of the available information. We had some data from questionnaires, but this was of doubtful validity. We had the evidence of who people spent time with as an indicator of personal relationships, and information from members of staff, and sometimes from relatives and friends. We also devised a flow-chart to guide our decision-making, which had criteria that someone would need to meet to be considered for the project. For this first house, the person would have to be:

1. Male for the reasons already given;
2. Physically fit. This was because there was no ground floor bedroom and the stairs were steep, also the shops were not very near;
3. They would need to be continent, as the house did not have facilities for 'foul' laundry;
4. They would have to be willing to take their medication;
5. They should be able to carry out basic self-care;

6. They should want to leave the hospital, or at least not be strongly opposed to the idea.

A set of inclusion criteria was chosen so that the first house would be relatively straightforward and so that the experience we gained would allow us to deal with more difficult problems later on. Having established that a person generally fitted these criteria we went on to consider their social network. If there was someone they were close to who could move out with them, that would be arranged. If their friend did not fit the criteria we would try and give them the option of a placement where they could stay together, or they could go to separate placements. By this means, we arrived at about ten men who might be suitable. The next step was to guess at which group might best fit in with each other. In this way, by going over and over the list we arrived at the six people who we would approach.

Informing the potential tenants

Each person was approached individually with details of the house, sometimes with a photograph, sometimes with written material. As we had been around for some time, it did not come as a shock to anyone. Nevertheless, we did not underestimate the emotional impact on people who had been in the hospital for many years to finally be told that they were to move out. We told this first group about six months before we expected the house to open. From this we learned the crucial importance of timing, as the slippage of ten months added unnecessary stress and frustration to what was already a highly stressful experience.

Grouping the residents

The first time the patients were brought together to meet each other and to discuss the fact that they would be moving to the same house together appeared to be more worrying for the team members who had convened the meeting. It raised many difficult feelings, and the subsequent meetings proved invaluable in answering questions. Again the delays on the project made a difficult task harder.

The team members' reaction to this first meeting was instructive in that it suggested considerable anxiety about what we were asking the patients to do. On the face of it, offering them a place in a pleasant house should be something one should feel little but pleasure about. In fact, we had become closely attuned to the sharp ambivalence people felt about the move and we were the harbingers of both good and bad news. It was not going to be easy for them to move out and we knew it.

Residents' visits to house

As the house progressed, visits were arranged so that the future tenants could choose their rooms and pick the colours for the wallpaper, carpets and other interior decor. These visits were of equal benefit for the team as for the tenants as the long months of planning with nothing to show for it were depressing, and to see real bricks and mortar lifted the spirits. On one visit, one person went into his room and shut the door and lay down on the floor (as there was no furniture yet). When someone knocked he did not reply as he had not had a room of his own for so long. These visits were also an opportunity to get to know the local area and were often combined with visits to other places.

We had lengthy discussions about informing the neighbours that a house was going to be opened and decided against such things as public meetings, or any sort of formal consultation. I made a postal survey of the pilot *'Care in the Community Programmes'* and it seemed from it that the best course was personal approaches to the immediate neighbours across the garden fence. This we have found has worked well, but depends on the project being well managed and being in the right area. Around this time we accompanied the residents to choose their furniture. This was organized rather well by the store in question who showed us round in a very pleasant manner, and laid on coffee and biscuits for us afterwards. The choice was rather limited and it was a mistake to have done a deal of this sort, despite the discount. The last house was able to shop around with its own budget and obtained a substantially improved range. During the phase when things became more real, we noticed that some of the future tenants became noticeably more anxious, and more individual support was needed at this time.

Recruiting staff

A training and recruitment group had been meeting since 1987 to organize the job descriptions, induction programme and other aspects of the personnel issues for the new service, and two resettlement team members were also members of this group. The staff for the project were recruited about two months before the opening date. We had taken advice that there should be enough time for the staff to get themselves together as a coherent team before starting shifts in the house. We were also advised that this time should not be too long so that they would develop patterns of work that were inappropriate for support work, which might have happened if they spent too much time in the hospital environment. The strategy favoured experienced/qualified house managers and unqualified support staff.

Training

The team, together with the training officer who started work with us from his post in the Learning Difficulties Care Group, designed the induction programme. The structure of the training was for the staff to spend some time in the hospital meeting the tenants and getting a feel for how they had been living. There were teaching sessions in Camberwell covering the following areas:

1. The structure of the services;
2. The history of Cane Hill;
3. A session describing the people moving in;
4. The role of the support worker;
5. Safety policies and procedures;
6. Medication policies and practices;
7. Social psychiatry;
8. Transition shock;
9. Useful approaches from psychology;
10. Social integration and imagery;
11. Individual programme planning;
12. Clinical services and social work;
13. Challenging behaviour — defining the challenge;
14. What skills were needed and how to get them;
15. Staying involved;
16. Team building;
17. Mental Health Act;
18. Household policies and procedures;
19. Service user's perspective;
20. Video 'We're Not Mad We're Angry'; and
21. Managing yourself as a support worker.

The other aspect of the work during the induction was to become familiar with the house and its environs. To ensure that the furniture was delivered on time (which is another story!) and to stock up the house with the things needed to run it. The consultant had approached the Family Practitioners Committee (now the Family Health Services Authority) at this point to find out the GP practice the tenants would be registering with. He visited the GPs personally, which went down very well and is to be recommended. This, together with the visit of a nurse from the team and the house manager with a clinical summary of each person, set up substantial long-lasting relationships between the GP service and the houses.

As there were eight staff for the house it was important to take care to introduce the residents individually and not to overwhelm them with the entire team descending on the ward at once. This was also a potentially tricky time for relationships with the hospital staff who may have felt that these young, casually dressed people were not competent to take over from them. Perhaps the support workers would regard the hospital staff as 'burnt out institutionalized has-beens'. Whatever the feelings it was an interaction that needed managing by the team and again it would have been better to have had more time.

Saying goodbye and moving in

Organizing the final stage of the move was very important, and again most of the work for this fell to the nurses. They had given every tenant a photograph album that had been filled up over the past few months with pictures of the hospital. We all felt it was important to acknowledge that the life people had been living in the hospital had positive memories. At a recent presentation, one nurse, Sally Mill, described the emotionally laden process of leaving for one person. All the patients had to collect papers from the general office, and this particular person saw his war medals for the first time since his admission in 1942. For others it was the sight of marriage certificates and death certificates that brought things back. It was a powerful and emotionally stirring experience. We were determined that there would be a dignified and respectful goodbye and people were helped to visit their favourite staff. The John Hutchinson Centre organized a party. Staff reactions were mixed; some were in tears, some could not be bothered to get up from the other side of the ward. For these staff, there was a strong feeling that they were watching something happen to them as well, something over which they had no control. The house staff at the other end had prepared a meal, which the men had chosen earlier. One man ate two dinners and was particularly taken with the 'real' potatoes as he had only had 'smash' at the hospital.

The use of the private and voluntary placements service

The placements service became one of the major strands of the resettlement strategy. It was not without its controversies, however. There had been a long-standing concern that patients were being trapped in hospital beds using up resources because of lack of alternative accommodation. Resistance on political grounds from the Local Authorities made placement in the private sector problematic as social workers were reluctant to be involved. A local initiative on the medical and physical handicap side had demonstrated that the use of this sector could:

> '...when carefully used and monitored...provide care for the elderly and young handicapped of a high standard. Most people relocated have settled well and prefer their new, more homely environment to prolonged stay in a hospital bed.'
>
> *(Jones and Golding,1986)*

They also pointed out that the cost 'to the State of private nursing home care was found to be half that of a hospital bed'.

The Placements Officer of the resettlement team had the remit to place as many patients as possible from Cane Hill as quickly as possible. This challenge exemplified the two elements of the strategy: (a) the need to find suitable alternative care and accommodation, as that provided at the hospital was deteriorating; and (b) and sometimes more importantly, to keep down costs and maximize income. An account of this service is given elsewhere (Booker *et al.*, 1989). It is briefly worth stating that a move to the private sector is no less an emotional experience and we found that several people became depressed after the move, so the follow-up provided by the team was important in maintaining continuity. The preparation of people to move was taken no less seriously for this group than for the people moving to the houses, although it sometimes happened with a shorter time scale.

The high-support house

The hostel was renamed the 'high-support house' and was opened in March 1992. It has places for ten people and work is in progress with the future residents as I write. They are generally in the younger age group and are competent in many ways; indeed, some of them have been keen to leave for some time. It has been hard for them to see people leaving for the other houses while they remain stuck in the hospital. Paradoxically, as the time to move out approaches they too are finding it difficult and we are not underestimating the emotional impact on them as with the others. The team is now operating on a consultancy basis to Hexagon Housing Association who won the tender competition to manage the house. This has freed us up to concentrate on the work in the hospital and avoid much of the policy development, job description and personnel matters, to our great relief. We feel this will be a very demanding service to run, thus the clinical team will continue to provide input to the house.

'Challenging behaviour'

A group of people were mentioned in the strategy in rather vague terms... 'There are a number of clients who present special difficulties and who must be planned for separately.' This included people who have been living in a locked ward for many years and for whom we still have inadequate information about how they may function in other settings. We have employed four psychology graduates for one year, specifically to work with this group so we can get a very detailed picture of their needs and can design some appropriate services. We have failed rather badly in devising good community-based services for this group and it may reflect the unresolved ideological differences that we have failed here. We have both capital and revenue, so we cannot blame that. At present we do not know what future these people have.

The so-called 'elderly graduates'

The rather odd title for this group refers to the fact that they have graduated to elderly status while in the hospital. As with the last group, these are people with great needs for services and will be the least well catered for. They were the group we had planned to accommodate in the purpose-built nursing home in the District. They are now being placed in the private sector and some are going to be living in West Park Hospital, one of the old asylums in the Epsom cluster.

The final phase of run-down

By April 1991, there were 17 patients in the Camberwell group left in the hospital. All the patients in the dementia service were placed in the private sector as there were worries about care standards. At this time, the facilities of the hospital were disappearing. The John Hutchinson Centre had now closed giving people the feeling that there would soon be nothing left. The management made a great effort to maintain morale during this period, planning such things as an event to commemorate the hospital's history.

RESETTLEMENT TEAM INVOLVEMENT IN OTHER SERVICE DEVELOPMENTS IN CAMBERWELL

The work programme

The strategy contained proposals for a sheltered work programme, as none was available in the East Lambeth sector of the District. A research project to evaluate the needs for such a service was commissioned after the British Institute of Industrial Therapy was approached by the team consultant in May 1987. The research proposed a series of interlinked work units based on catering, woodwork and painting and decorating. We have since obtained funding from the Department of the Environment and have purchased a property and at the time of writing the builders were on site. A company called the Southside Rehabilitation Association has been set up to run it, and I am the Chairman. It is likely that another work programme called 'Sweepers' being developed by the Maudsley group will join our organization. It will have something in the region of 30 to 45 places.

The social club

This project, described as 'low key' in the strategy, is now open and team members have been actively involved in its development. This programme went to tender and the Mental After-Care Association has a contract with Camberwell Health District to provide the service. It will be attempting to develop a club-house style, with members rather than patients, clients or other titles. The members can attend for as long as they feel the need to. There is a café on site. The people living in the houses will be encouraged to join.

The advocacy service

This element was included in the strategy partly as a consequence of the Health Authority's commitment to equal opportunities, a policy for which it had just published when we were working on the strategy. We used the £20 000 per year to fund a few groups who were able to provide advocacy or similar types of support. In the long term, we have funded Lambeth

Forum, a consumer group, which has started up a tenants' association for the people living in the houses. The Forum and groups related to it are growing at a great pace; they represent the growing confidence and sophistication of the consumer movement, which is greatly to be welcomed.

PROGRESS REVIEW

Review of the functioning of the resettlement team

In reviewing the functioning of the resettlement team during the years we have worked together, it is striking how we have managed to remain committed to each other and to the process. The team has had successes and failures. There have been times when we have been very angry with each other and yet have kept the coherence of the team. One principal reason for this is that when things appear to be falling apart, which happens from time to time, we take a day out together to consider our objectives. We have had about ten of these during the course of the past five years. Some have been very uncomfortable affairs as they draw attention to the gaps in the team's functioning. We are explicit that the days are to deal with both emotional as well as practical issues. If a team member does not feel listened to they can raise it then. Another useful mechanism was a weekly support group, with no outside facilitator. This was used, in general, to identify who was that week's external reason for problems. Once identified, we were able to enjoy ourselves before coming back to our own shortcomings.

Finally, there was genuine respect within the team for each other's ideas, despite strongly differing views on the nature of the problems of the clients we were seeking to support.

The lessons to be learned

The lessons from this experience fall into several categories and apply at different levels and in different areas. These are considered in turn.

The process of closing Cane Hill

The running-down of the hospital was a managerial nightmare. There was no single agency with the authority to make things happen. In services where the hospital was in the catchment area of the provider District the issues were less sharp but, in this case, the hospital was managed extra-territorially by Bromley on behalf of other Authorities. The Regional Health Authority had a nominal leadership role, but either chose not to or was incapable of exercising it. The need to ensure that there was close co-ordination between the contraction of the hospital and the developing community services was crucial, but almost impossible with the structure within which we were working.

There is some sense in adopting the Fulbourne Hospital model in Cambridge, in which a long-term view was taken whereby the community facilities were gradually brought on-line while maintaining the hospital as a viable service, however imperfect. In time, the hospital may be no longer needed, and that will be the time to let it go.

The skills and experience of workers

The skills of the team members were discussed earlier. The criticisms of the team would be that there should have been experience in the areas that were missing in our team, particularly in the workings of the mental hospital. Effective collaboration with the institution is essential to a smooth resettlement programme. In addition, the effectiveness of the consumer group locally suggests that a team member with experience as a service user would be of great value.

In addition, we also were carrying out far too many roles and the task we were asked to take on was too large. The idea that the planning of the service should be informed by people who knew the patients was a good one and ought to be repeated, but the scope of the work required of the team should be clearly demarcated to avoid the overcommitment we experienced.

Models of service provision and ideology

Ideological issues are central to the way services develop. We have struggled to form a synthesis between social psychiatry and notions from normalization theory. We have had some success in this but it is a constant problem, and the two models are probably not reconcilable. It is not helped by the more extreme or vulgar versions of both having articulate advocates. The psychiatric model will tend to be overcoercive and the normalization model underestimates the degree of handicap. There is much work to be done in this area and we do not debate it in the team sufficiently openly. It affects the possible options, for example, for the people in the so-called 'challenging behaviour' group and has meant that imaginative solutions, such as those proposed by Taylor *et al.* in 1987, find little support. Again it is possible that the consumer model, which requires good quality services and which aims to ensure that whatever the model, it meets people's needs, will have much to contribute. One particular area in which it has become problematic is in supporting people living in the houses who behave in socially frightening or embarrassing ways. Ideology apart, unless we are able to support such people in these settings, we will be priced out of the market.

Finance and fine words

Finance had been the main driving force behind the closure plan and is very important. It is true to say that we were not idealistic at the start of the process but we underestimated the over-riding importance of money. One cannot go wrong overestimating the importance of finance. Since finance is so important there is a duty to get the figures right, and in our experience they rarely were. This is not to say that the managers do not have feelings about this as the following anecdote illustrates. I was driving back from the hospital with a member of our management team and sharing with him the fact that one of the patients had died a couple of days earlier. I noticed a bit of a commotion in the passenger seat and it turned out that he had felt two feelings simultaneously; one was that a death was £25 000 more for the Camberwell services, always strapped for cash. Equally strong was the feeling of sadness at another person dying before getting out of Cane Hill.

The impact of the NHS changes with the introduction of the internal market will radically alter all future closure exercises, and it is going to be difficult to generalize from the experience in this area as funding mechanisms are likely to be totally different.

A final area we have learned is that any voluntary organization that is set up to provide services should have very robust financial control mechanisms or things will get rapidly into a mess and the consumers will suffer.

A balanced service system

A range of services is needed if it is to be truly comprehensive and the strategy attempted to design one which at least could claim to have some comprehensiveness. The loss of the nursing home was a major blow that distorted the outcome substantially. Team members feel that we have let people down having told them that we were getting places for them in Camberwell and now not coming up with the goods. However, it is clear that supported housing is a feasible and useful component of the system. The high-support house is the next level up and it will be interesting to see how it functions. It will have to take quite disturbed people, since it will be an expensive facility. It is definitely community-based, however, and situated away from a hospital site, so it is quite experimental in some ways. The next level of security above this has not been developed but is likely to be on a hospital site, unless we can come up with more imaginative solutions.

In our experience, we were unable to plan the service in sufficient collaboration with our colleagues in the Maudsley Hospital. If we had, we may have done things differently.

The private sector

The huge expansion of this area of service provision has had a major impact on the way the service developed. It is still to be evaluated, but I have major concerns about its use on such a large scale. As noted in Booker *et al.* (1989), the American evidence is not good on the use of this type of service:

'The failure to have evaluated adequately the effect of discharging hundreds of thousands of chronically mentally ill patients from large public mental hospitals has been a major defect in the conduct of public policy.'

(Braun et al., 1981)

Consequences of the move for the residents

One way to understand the overall outcome for the residents is to consider the common experiences of people who are subjected to social devaluation, the so-called 'wounds' most recently formulated by Wolfensberger (1987) and described in Figure 1.9. The risks that people who are on the receiving

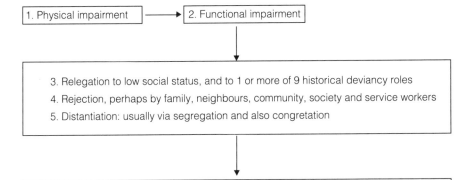

Figure 1.9 The most common 'wounds' of devalued (and especially handicapped) people.

end of this process of social devaluation face are many (and the Cane Hill residents fall into this group) but include being moved around so that social relationships are broken, and links with familiar places severed. There is a loss of autonomy over your life, and you tend to be treated as one of a mass rather than an individual. You tend to be grouped with others who are also viewed by society as less worthy than average, so you are stigmatized very strongly. People who are devalued are kept poor, and their talents are often wasted. As pointed out recently (Wolfensberger, 1990; Abrahams, 1990), for many people the process is so severe that it leads to their lives being shortened or their being actually killed.

Of the original 117 people nearly 40% have died. This mostly reflects the age of the people, and we have no evidence that there has been here an increased number of people dying as a result of the moves. This will be finally known when the process is finished. For the remaining people, about a quarter are now living or will be living in supported accommodation through the projects that we have specifically developed. For those living in the supported housing, many of the 'wounds' still apply.

For those who have moved into the private and voluntary sector, again approximately a quarter of the original residents, I have concerns about their situation. In general, they are living in comfortable surroundings, and there is no doubt that in that respect things have improved. However, in other aspects such as the lack of purposeful activity, lack of friendship networks, segregated settings and many others in the 'wounds' matrix, they are as badly off as in the hospital. Furthermore, all the people moving out are in some ways worse off than when they were in the hospital. In the hospital there were daily activities, not necessarily very relevant, but they were there. In many nursing homes they are simply not available and, with financial constraints, they are not likely to increase. For a small group, something over 10%, the future is in another mental hospital and, for those, the issues for which we originally undertook the resettlement programme remain.

The challenge is to develop ways of securing positive futures for people who rely on mental health services. In the words of one American worker in this field, 'we are at the limit of what we can rent'. From the experience of this closure programme, the future would seem to lie in improving the service's competence in helping people make personal commitments to each other, and one major route to this is through the user movement. This movement is enhancing the status of people with mental health problems — they are becoming people to know! Secondly, communities have become de-skilled by the process that has shut away those with mental health problems — out of sight, out of mind. As they return, or remain in their own homes, there is a major effort required to ensure that helpful responses are organized from these communities by utilizing networks of friends and relatives and voluntary groups and that these are adequately resourced.

Social policy shifts have been useful here in changing the focus away from the institution towards more ordinary settings, but to be effective money must follow the vision. For those most disabled, this challenge is the greatest since they remain, in large measure, hidden away from mainstream society.

Models of provision that allow for safety for all concerned but which are neither punitive nor segregating are the most urgent need for services to develop and it is here that we have made least progress. However, much energy is going into developing provision in this area and this may yet yield dividends.

REFERENCES

Abrahams, R. (1990) Deathmaking — The evidence and trends in Britain and Europe. *Changes*, **8**, (4), 294–303.

Andrews, C. T. (1978) *The Dark Awakening: A History of St Lawrence's Hospital*. St Lawrence's Hospital Publishers, Bodmin.

Booker, D., Holloway, F., Mill, S., Siddle, K. and Wilson,. (1989) Private placements and the chronically mentally ill. *Health Service Journal*, 20–25.

Braun, P., Kochansky, G., Shapiro, R., Greenberg, S., Gudeman, J., Johnson, S. and Shore, M. F. (1981) Overview: De-institutionalization of psychiatric patients, a critical review of outcome studies. *American Journal of Psychiatry*, **138**, 736–749.

Brost, M.M. and Johnson, T. Z. (1982) *Getting to Know You: One Approach to Service Assessment and Planning for Individuals with Disabilities*. Wisconsin Coalition for Advocacy and New Concepts for the Handicapped Foundation Inc., Wisconsin, USA.

Camberwell Resettlement Team (1988) *From Cane Hill to Camberwell: A Progress Report*.

Cane Hill Research Team (1990) *Evaluating the Closure of Cane Hill Hospital: Plans for Residential Services and the Long-stay Population*. Research & Development in Psychiatry, London.

Clifford, P. (1986) *Cane Hill Hospital Patients' Needs Survey*. NUPRD, London.

Commissioners in Lunacy reports 1890–1920. Reports on Cane Hill and related hospitals.

Gowler, D. and Parry, G. (1979) Professionalism and its discontents. *New Forum*, **5**, (4), 54–56.

Holloway, F. (1990) Caring for people: a critical review of government policy for the mentally ill. *Psychiatric Bulletin*, **14**, 641–5.

Hospital Advisory Service (1978) *Cane Hill Visit Report No. HAS/SWS/ (78) MI 252*. HAS, London.

Jones, K. and Golding A. M. B (1986) *After Hospital: A study of long-term psychiatric patients in York*, Department of Social Policy and Social Work, The University of York, York.

King, D. (1988) Replacing mental hospitals with better services. In: S. Ramon (ed.) *Psychiatry in Transition*, Pluto Press, London.

Ovretviet, J. (1986) *Organization of multidisciplinary community teams*, Health Services Centre Working Paper, Brunel University, Uxbridge.

Peck E. (1985) Planning not platitudes. *Health and Social Services Journal*, 78–79.

South East Thames Regional Health Authority, SETRHA (1987) *A Service in Transition — Priorities for the Development of Local Mental Health Services to Replace Large Mental Hospitals in the South East Thames Region*. SERTHA, London.

Taylor, S. J., Racino, J. A., Knoll, J. A. and Luftiyya, Z. (1987) *The nonrestrictive environment: on community integration for people with the most severe disabilities*, Human Policy Press, Syracuse.

Thorneycroft, G. (1988) *Preliminary Report on Baseline Data from Friern and Claybury Hospitals, Team for the Assessment of Psychiatric Hospitals*, NETRHA, London

Wainwright, A. (1986) *Thoughts on Cane Hill*. (Unpublished)

Wainwright, A. (1987) *Problems encountered in the transitional period between the closure of Cane Hill Hospital and the development of successor services*. (Unpublished.)

Wainwright, A., Holloway, F. and Brugha, T. (1988) Day care in an inner city area. In: A. Lavender and F. Holloway (eds.) *Community Care in Practice*, Wiley, Chichester.

Wainwright, A. and Lindley, P. (1991) Normalization training: conversion or commitment. In: Brown H. and Smith, H. *Normalization: A Reader for the Nineties*, Routledge, London.

Walk, A. (Various dates) Papers on the History of Psychiatry: a collection of unpublished writings together with a record of published papers and other printed items by the ex Medical Superintendent of Cane Hill. Collected by his wife, Margaret L. Walk.

Watts, F. and Bennett, D. (1983) Management of the staff team. In: Watts, F. and Bennett, D. (eds) *Theory and Practice of Psychiatric Rehabilitation*, Wiley, Chichester.

Wolfensberger, W. (1983) Social role valorization: a proposed new term for the principle of normalization. *Mental Retardation*, **21**, 234–239.

Wolfensberger, W. (1987) *The New Genocide of Handicapped and Afflicted People*. Syracuse University, Syracuse, New York.

Wolfensberger, L. (1990) A most critical issue: Life or Death. *Changes*, **8**, (1) 63–73.

2

Planning after a closure decision: The case of the North East Thames Regional Health Authority

DYLAN TOMLINSON

THE CONTEXT

Much attention has been given to the de-institutionalization process in the USA and Italy (Ramon, 1983; Samson, 1990, Tomlinson, 1991).

In the USA

In the USA, cost containment has been commonly identified as the main reason for the large-scale reduction achieved in the in-patient population of mental hospitals. The Federal Government has attempted to pass the costs of mental health across to the States, which have been unwilling to raise local taxes to meet those costs. The Kennedy administration launched mental health initiatives that were to lead to the creation of more than 500 community mental health centres, and to national optimism about what the mental health services could offer. However, these initiatives did not lead to the development of a securely funded nationwide network of health centres. The intention was that Federal finance would only be necessary to pump prime the centres. The latter were to be eventually self-funding from private or public insurance contributions. This meant that, to survive, the new system would have to attract patients with resources. Few of the residents of mental hospitals, once resettled in the community, would be able to bring such resources. Likewise, the substantial minority of America's poor not eligible for State medical support and not covered by employer's health insurance schemes would be unable to do so. While long-stay patients were being discharged from the USA's large hospitals, the community systems that would replace them were thus being starved of funds. Nevertheless, there are less pejorative judgements in the literature on the changes in mental health care in the USA. One would suggest that a national obsession with securing the civil liberty of the individual has resulted in the collective social rights of uncompetitive and marginal groups such as the mentally ill being neglected.

In Italy

In Italy, radical politics has been held to account for de-institutionalization (Ramon, 1983). Communitarian and anti-authoritarian principles of new services have stressed the rights of long-stay patients to be re-admitted to the civil society, to occupy housing of good standard and to be able to take up employment. In effect, to have their social status upgraded to the point at which it is broadly equivalent to that of their therapists.

In Britain

In this context, the startling decision of the North East Thames Regional Health Authority (NETRHA) to close all its six mental hospitals, and to target two of them for closure within the ten-year period from 1983 to 1993, seems highly unusual (NETRHA, 1983). There was only some injection of extra funding to the mental illness sector, which was initially 9% additional revenue to the revenue that was being spent on the two hospitals targeted for early closure. At the same time, £50 million was set aside for the construction, acquisition and conversion costs of developing community units. However this fell far short of what NETRHA's officers later referred to, with some acuity, as the 'aspirations' of the planners in the constituent district authorities of the region.

When beginning a study of the implementation of the NETRHA decision, early in 1985, I was struck by the vision and commitment to the closure policy of top Regional Health Authority CRHA officers. Amid a mass of feasibility data and analysis of trends that heralded the final decision on closure, it was clear that, at a subjective level, the RHA's officers simply felt that it was unacceptable to continue to provide services from the decaying large hospitals.

After visiting the two hospitals due for closure during their deliberation, they had been dismayed by the appalling conditions in which staff were struggling to work. While the scandal factor has been a major impetus to achieving the change away from mental hospitals, scandals have a habit of coming and going, in between more pressing national concerns such as wars. The public's ability to tolerate a certain level of scandalous conditions is difficult to judge. RHA officers might have been committed to the closure in 1983, but by 1986 those who had developed the policy had all left the employment of the Authority. Without their subjective commitment to underpin the objective assessment of the feasibility of closure, would the will to push the policy through be lost?

When the decision to close the two hospitals was taken, there were more than 1700 in-patient beds in them. Each hospital served districts in London itself. To enable their closure, community placements were to be provided for all long-stay residents as part of a large-scale, bed-for-bed hospital 'reprovision' programme. These placements were planned to range from hostels sited on the periphery of general hospital sites for the most dependent patients, through staffed group homes and nursing homes for those of average dependency, to independent flats for the most able minority. Housing associations, voluntary organizations, and local authorities would collaborate with the hospital managing authorities in bringing about the new services.

Since these hospitals served inner-city and deprived areas of London there was much anxiety about the effects of replacing them with alternative services. Indeed, at an early point in the planning process, it was decided only to partially close one of them, retaining part of the site to serve the population of the borough lying nearest to the hospital. The logic behind this was to provide a 'failsafe' position such that if, as critics argued, many ex-patients found it difficult to cope outside the hospitals, the possibility of keeping a 'mini' Friern Hospital in perpetuity would still be open.

However, RHA officers cautioned that if the land value of the retained parcel of the site became very great, then this failsafe position would be reviewed. It was argued that the RHA's mental health goals for the whole region might then be better advanced by moving off the site entirely. Without the cash from the sale of the whole site, there would be ultimately that much less capital money to spread around. Although the £50 million mentioned above was set aside for the development costs of the new community facilities required to close the two hospitals, the NETRHA was also busy supporting new general hospitals in the traditionally under-resourced Essex areas of the region, such as Southend. This put the hospital site, which was situated in a valuable residential zone, under some pressure as an asset that would need to be sold at the earliest opportunity. Indeed, in 1989, such had the funding difficulties of the NETRHA become, that the feasibility of closing the hospital 18 months before the 1993 deadline, in order to vacate the site, was investigated.

As a result of the anxiety and outright opposition to the RHA's closure policy among clinical 'opinion leaders' at the other hospital, Regional officers agreed to commission an evaluation of the entire ten-year progress of the resettlement of patients. The staff there were assured that if the evaluators found, in the interim, that results were poor, then the RHA would rethink the entire dispersal policy. In 1985, TAPS (Team for Assessment of Psychiatric Services) was set up as an independent unit, with an initial grant from the King's Fund, as well as Department of Health and Social Security and RHA funding, to carry out this task. The author is a founder member of the team (Tomlinson, 1988; TAPS, 1988).

THE BEGINNINGS OF CLOSURE

Motivation

Are mental hospital closures part of a government strategy to sell off the NHS estate and cash in on community care? My own research suggests that this hypothesis should be treated with extreme circumspection. It can be argued that there are five stimuli for mental hospital closures in England and Wales. These are: (a) government guidelines; (b) professional value choices; (c) the performance and accountability review system by which Health Authorities' progress against targets is measured; (d) mental health administration issues; and (e) pressure from concerned groups such as Community Health Councils and MIND.

Four of these stimuli were relatively absent in the case of these two hospitals. There was no Central Government edict forcing the controlling Regional Health Authority to select these, or indeed any, hospitals for closures. Rather, central government was advising the Regional Health Authority to move cautiously toward community services. Many observers complained of the vacillation of the then DHSS, which allowed a demonstration closure project at Powick Hospital in Worcester to proceed over a leisurely 20 years, while the asylums continued to crumble around the country, and the revolutionary changes in Italy and the USA reverberated. Government circulars gave *carte blanche* to the 'do nothing' option: provided any asylum was situated reasonably near to its catchment population it could continue to serve, paradoxically, within a network of new local, devolved, community services. By following this policy, the Government ensured that plausible arguments could be put forward at both hospitals for their retention on this ground alone.

A rather appealing argument about closure of asylums would be that the Conservative Government arrived in 1979 and rapidly set about their dissolution. However, this too easily overlooks the proposals introduced by the Labour Government in 1975 for a District General Hospital-centred network of services (DHSS, 1975). While some mental hospitals were to 'continue in use for many years', joint planning was to achieve the 'early replacement' of those 'whose physical conditions and geographical location are likely to provide the greatest handicap'. Having just experienced the so-called 'fiscal crisis' of 1974, and envisaging only marginal growth in public expenditure, the Government was careful to note that the development of a new pattern of service would take many years to achieve.

In political terms then, it is difficult to see the targeting of ageing mental hospitals for closure as manifesto-led. Certainly, the corporate strength of the medical and, to a much lesser extent, that of the nursing professions, would serve to ensure that care structures for people with mental illness would be difficult to erode. Although psychiatrists could hardly be seen as a group whose mouths were stuffed with gold by the NHS, nevertheless their role would be important in the negotiation of specific closures.

The mental health issue can be defined as a 'strategic low' for a government, in contrast to Palmer's 'strategic highs' such as regulation of the oil industry, to which Central Government attaches importance (Palmer, 1985). So long as Central Government does not become too deeply interested in mental health, it is likely that the providers — the caring professions — will continue to set the agenda.

Neither of the two lower-level district authorities that were responsible for day-to-day management had set itself the task of closure. This, to some extent, reflected the immaturity of District Health Authorities, since they had only been created the year before closure was decided upon in 1982. Nor had the Regional Health Authority set them any annual bed-reduction targets against which they could be monitored. There had been no lobby from the professional care staffs to achieve rundown: rather they were much divided on the issue, as will be seen later. There was diffuse pressure from CHCs for admissions to the hospitals to stop, which particularly affected one hospital, but that did not stem from the basis of any special broad campaign. Rather, it came about because of bad publicity about abuses of patients or the conditions in which they were kept, which appeared in the Press from time to time. *The Sun* newspaper ran a story of around 2000 words in 1978 making allegations of abuse on a particular ward (Tomlinson, 1991).

At a national level, the voluntary organizations took up positions characterized by much diversity on the question of the future of asylums.

To what then can we attribute the North East Thames programme?

The drive behind Friern and Claybury Hospitals closure can mostly be attributed to mental health administration issues. Three in particular may be singled out:

1. An important event for the development of social services and other related services such as health was the publication of the Barclay Report in 1982. This was, in effect, a Government prospectus for the future organization of social work. The big change was that the client was no longer to be seen in isolation as a problem person, but as one whose fate and characteristics were bound together with the family, the neigh-bourhood and other friendship networks. The role of social workers was to lend support to these 'natural' kinship and neighbouring networks of people who were vulnerable, so that they could be steered through crises. Social services would be organized on a patch basis to undertake this work. With hindsight, we are aware today that the recommendations of this report were largely ignored by local authorities. Health authorities were at the time moving toward similar goals as the social services authorities, and were given a further stimulus by Barclay. The culmination of many years of debate in nursing was the Cumberlege report of 1988, in which the DHSS suggested that 'neighbourhood nursing' was a 'focus for care'. Asylums covering large catchment areas were simply dinosaurs due for extinction in this new pattern of health-care coverage (Barclay, 1982; Cumberledge, 1988).

2. Several reorganizations of the NHS, especially in 1974 and 1982, had been designed to strengthen the management of the organization, moving away from the 'great and the good' model of the hospital as the

core unit of health care. The new expenditure constraints, together with the technological, social and demographic challenges facing the NHS placed too great an expectation on the capacities of lay, unelected, non-executive Hospital Board members. The trend was toward making Health Authorities more administratively accountable to Central Government for the development of local services. Mental hospitals were being subjected to the same drive to strengthen centralized managerial control and would no longer be fixed stars in the firmament.

3. The dilapidation of the asylum buildings, constructed originally at a cost to the rate-payer, but which no local authority would have the will to restore. None of the new District Health Authorities had the power to raise funds for such restoration. At a very early stage in NETRHA's history (1976), its managers recognized that there was a choice between either putting resources into community developments or putting them into the asylums.

The *raison d'etre* of the District Health Authorities was the District General Hospital, seen as the nucleus of care from which all services should radiate to smaller satellite District bases. The two hospitals, by their very existence, challenged the notion of General Hospital psychiatry being at the centre of the service. The major obstacle to General Hospital take-over was that the psychiatric units within them were not designed to provide long-term care on a large scale and did not usually provide the range of therapeutic activities that the mental hospitals offered to their elderly residents. It is worthy of note that, even at the time of writing (April 1991), a TAPS study that the author is involved in has identified a dozen patients who have been resident in either hospitals since before 1930. Clearly, such patients have considerably more experience of mental health care than anyone working or living in a General Hospital environment.

Was it humane?

Was it humane to uproot the elderly long-stay population of the asylums just to clear the grounds for sale and provide for the funding of new services? Would nursing home, hostel or group-home placements be suitable for this category of institution resident? The proposed partial closure of the hospital allowed for some of the group, at least, to stay behind.

One of the great misconceptions is that the closures have been brought about by psychiatrists unlocking all the doors and pushing patients out into any and every available type of bed-and-breakfast accommodation. It is true that clinicians had been at the forefront of the efforts to get people out of hospital. There had been various drives to get the in-patient population down (for example, with the Islington Division at Friern in the mid-1970s), which resulted in a considerable reduction in the number of long-stay residents. Claybury, on the other hand, as the Regional Medical Officer commented, still enjoyed to some extent living under the halo of the therapeutic community for which it had been acclaimed in the 1960s and 1970s (Bromley, 1984).

Was it too great a challenge?

However, the position in the early 1980s appeared to be much more one of stagnation. An argument often advanced by the clinicians to account for this state-of-affairs was that the resident patients remaining in the asylums were too severely disabled to be moved out. The theory was that the rehabilitation of those remaining was just too great a challenge. Most were simply not 'rehabilitation material', in contrast to those who had left the hospital in the previous two decades. The resident population was predominantly made up of patients diagnosed as suffering from schizophrenia, often labelled 'harder to place' for such reasons as being arsonists, verbally or physically abusive, or perpetually at risk of self harm. It was argued that this population had been subjected to various unsuccessful attempts at resettlement down the years. In this process, patients had either not 'stayed the course' outside hospital or been repeatedly rejected as candidates for resettlement by agencies providing community placements (Furlong, 1985). On the basis of this experience, many psychiatrists at these hospitals were extremely sceptical about the chances of the wholesale resettlement of the asylum population being achievable.

This perspective was well summed up in two articles that appeared in the English psychiatrists' in-house *Monthly Bulletin* during 1985 (Fagin, 1985; Furlong, 1985). One of the articles was written by Fagin, a Consultant at Claybury who, in a sense, carried on the tradition of experimental innovation at that hospital, having played a major role in establishing a community mental health centre in the catchment area. Drawing on a period of study in the USA, his article interpreted 'the writing on the wall' for the Victorian asylums, which the American experience of de-institutionalization conveyed. The other article in the monthly bulletin was written by Furlong, a Consultant at Friern Hospital, who, as Chair of its Medical Committee, had been a spokesperson in the debates that followed the NETRHA closure decision. She questioned whether the closure of mental hospitals was either practicable or desirable.

Fagin's is the more optimistic of the two articles with respect to the process of closure, citing evidence from the USA that showed that well-planned alternatives to mental hospital are feasible to operate. Nevertheless he points out that the context for such changes is one where the public hospitals 'are still the only choice of facility when it comes to socially deviant, disruptive individuals' and where 'issues of violence involve 60% of admissions, with hospital patient populations becoming skewed toward this type of patient.'

Examining the prevalence of nursing homes as an alternative to mental hospitals in the USA, Fagin reports that this can be explained by the fact that insurance services do not cover many of the community facilities required by discharged patients.

Furlong, from a base barely ten miles across London from that of Fagin, argues for the retention of large psychiatric hospital facilities for the most disabled patients. She argues this on two grounds. Firstly, because Government assumptions about the proportion of remaining hospital residents who are capable of living 'ordinary lives in the community' are falsely high. This is because they extrapolate from knowledge about the dependency of the patient population that was resident in the asylums in the 1970s, many of whom had long since been discharged. Secondly, Furlong suggests that the move to the community would be likely to have an adverse effect on a substantial number of patients. The resettlement of patients in tight-knit group homes would place too many socializing demands on those with chronic schizophrenia. At the same time, the asocial or apathetic condition of many of those falling into this diagnostic group was attributable, in some part, to the illness that they suffered from rather than institutionalization. Therefore moving patients into the community would hold little prospect of rehabilitation.

Was it casting off responsibility?

NETRHA was anxious to avoid being seen as closing hospitals in order to cast off responsibility for the remaining long-term patients. The worry was that if Furlong and her colleagues were right, subjecting the 'harder to place' population to an enforced resettlement could lead to a situation where, especially if staff were not wholly supportive of the moves, closure would be unpopular with patients and the general public. Apart from the psycho-political fall-out this might cause, there was the possibility of many 'ex-patients' simply absconding from their community placements because so many demands had been made on them in the new facilities. Many might move on to large hostels for the homeless in central London, where they would not have to be subjected to any psychiatric regime. These hostels already housed a considerable number of the homeless who were known to have received a hospital diagnosis of mental illness at one time or another. Easily accessible for interviews both to journalists and the opponents of community care alike, such refugees from enforced resettlement might easily become the 'Banquo's ghosts' in nightmares of Regional officers.

New community placements

For these reasons, it was agreed at an early stage in the closure process at the two hospitals that a special 'new' community placement would be provided for every resident in-patient. Where judged necessary by medical and nursing staff, this would provide the same level of care or a better level than had been provided by the hospital. The significance of this decision was that the NETRHA, in effect, accepted the psychiatrists' argument about the difficulty of resettlement. Patients transferred to the community would not be under any more pressure to leave the new forms of care than they had been to leave that of the mental hospital. The new community placements would be different from the 'run-of-the-mill' after-care facilities, such as group homes and supervised hostels, that social services and voluntary organizations had always provided. The latter were intended as half-way houses in the anticipated patient graduation back to 'ordinary' living, and were therefore temporary. However, the establishments that would replace the mental hospitals would be intended to provide permanent residences for those moving into them. This was recognition indeed of the likely difficulties in enabling the remaining patients to achieve a degree of 'normal life'.

In many ways, when the closure of these two hospitals is judged against those adopted elsewhere, the NETRHA's determination to create a discrete residential and day-care system to literally 're-provide' the services of the two hospitals was a bold and enlightened decision. Firstly, it ensured almost beyond dispute that a far higher quality of accommodation and environment would be provided in the community services than in the dilapidated 'backwards' of the asylum. Secondly, it ensured that the funding of mental health services, at least in terms of Regional Health Authority (but not necessarily District Health Authority) disbursement, would be maintained during a period when all other sectors of the NHS in London were suffering from the impact of the RAWP formula (i.e. the redistribution of resources from London to the rest of the country). Thirdly, it gave mental health a high profile and an opportunity for advancing the cause of decentralized, destigmatized, and integrated community services in a period when general social policy did not favour marginalized social groups such as people with mental illness.

Nevertheless, this decision inevitably had its downside, in that special residential and day-care facilities were to be set up under a mental health banner. This carried the added dangers of labelling and 'transinstitu-tionalization'. As already mentioned, the argument that the 1980s long-stay population in the asylums was far more chronic and difficult to resettle than the 1960s or 1970s populations was accepted by the RHA. In turn, those patients were consigned to chronicity. They had not been consulted on these decisions. Indeed, at that time, in 1983, it was hardly thought possible to engage in a process of consultation with resident patients.

Reaffirmation of chronicity
It may be noted here that the reaffirmation of chronicity grew out of the philosophy of the pioneer psychiatrists who shook the world of asylums by

opening the doors and setting up therapeutic communities in the late 1940s and 1950s. In their view, the chronic population would probably not benefit from new techniques and attempts to prevent patients from throwing all their social responsibilities onto the nursing staff and other carers. Indeed, they considered that institutionalization was probably the 'best outcome' for many of those they termed chronic (Martin, 1955). However, the pioneers clearly felt that the key was to prevent patients from becoming chronic. Without this chronic population having built up, there would be no reason for keeping asylums. This perception led to the virtues of asylums being seen later on as synonymous with protection of those with chronic conditions. These are Furlong's positive attributes, which can be contrasted, as in Table 2.1, with the negative attributes for the non-chronic population, outlined by Martin (1968), who was the physician superintendent at Claybury in the 1960s.

Table 2.1 Positive and negative aspects of institutions: an overview from Friern and Claybury pyschiatrists, 1955–1985

Positive aspects for a 'chronic' population (Furlong, 1985)	Negative aspects for a non-'chronic' population (Martin, 1955)
There is less potential for friction where patients have the space of the asylum grounds and large open-plan dormitories	People are relieved of their social and personal responsibilities on being admitted to hospital
The lack of volition of people with chronic conditions is likely to mean that they will have a continuing need to be organized	Organized recreation, occupational therapy and sheltered industrial therapy requires no effort on the part of the patients
There is a common experience of rejection by community agencies offering placements among the chronic mentally ill	Institutions offer protection from pressures in the community that should spur the patient to address his/her problems
People with schizophrenia do not necessarily benefit from closer contact with relatives, friends and others in the community outside hospital	Long-term patients lose 'objective' awareness of their social position while in hospital

Could it have been otherwise? Were medical and nursing staff in the mid-1980s really able to offer nothing more to the population judged chronic than their predecessors in the 1950s? This question could never be properly addressed in planning because of the message of rejection that psychiatrists and nurses felt was being strongly conveyed to them by the top-down process of decision-making (Garelick, 1988). Quite simply, as noted above, the care given in the asylums was seen by senior Health Authority staff as unacceptable. Arguments put forward in defence of the role of psychiatric hospitals were seen as protection of empires,ivory towers, sinecures and the dubious privilege of staff accommodation. In retrospect, too little consideration of this issue had been given in the 1975 blueprint, which simply stated that while plans were developing 'the staff of the mental hospitals ... should be kept fully in the picture.' (DHSS, 1975).

These, then, were the circumstances in which ward nursing staff were to implement the RHA's plans and prepare chronic institutionalized patients for a new life in the community. Predictably, a key problem in the devolution of Friern and Claybury hospital services to the community has been the lack of involvement of ward staff in their development (Towell and Macausland, 1988). That consultation with patients about the options for resettlement was not undertaken, reflects further this lack of engagement. Without the commitment of their carers, how could patients so used to having decisions made for them be interested in and motivated toward life outside the hospital? In large part, the closure decisions were taken by senior Regional Health Authority (RHA) and District Health Authority (DHA) officers, with the designs for alternatives not coming from within the hospitals. When closure has, in effect, been imposed on the hospitals from on high, it has obviously been more difficult for their managers to justify it, or to engineer from within a situation in which the more receptive staff are nurtured as leaders of the change, and patient advocates (McKee and Pettigrew, 1988). Where once the staff of institutions were the revolutionaries, developing therapeutic communities and encouraging patients to take back responsibility, they are now cast as the reactionaries. Planners and managers now have the solutions, not staff.

THE CONCEPTUAL AND MORAL UNDERPINNING OF THE PLANNED CLOSURE

Normalization interpreted

In a normalization programme, the task for the staff is about working with clients so that they can solve problems, take options and pursue valued activities. The objective is not to make clients do the same things as some normative social group that is the model. One cannot go to the normal-ization handbook and write out a prescription for a desired set of activities and tasks. The imminent tendency within statutory planning is to suppose that such prescription exists.

Renshaw identifies four elements within normalization:

Firstly, everyone has the basic human right to be accepted as a full member of society, to be treated as an individual, with dignity and respect, and with the

opportunity to exercise some choice and control over their own life. Secondly,
people with handicaps (or other demeaning conditions) start from a position of
disadvantage from which they require better than average circumstances to
bring them back to a point of equal opportunity. Thirdly, strong emphasis is
placed on encouragement and help for people with handicaps to improve their
skills and abilities. Fourthly, services should be planned to meet individual
needs, rather than individuals fitted to services.'

(Renshaw, 1985)

'Passing' system of normalization

Most people involved in planning services could subscribe readily to these
general principles, but few were aware that a system called 'passing' had
been developed with which to judge how 'normalizing' particular services
offered might be. Psychologists and some officers knowledgeable of the
field of mental handicap were familiar with the system, but those possess-
ing this knowledge constituted a tiny minority on the fringe. For this
reason, in the minds of most participants, normalization at a practical level
meant, crudely, introducing a normal environment and normal conditions
into 'reprovision' projects. It meant that patients, once in the community,
would do the same sort of things as everybody else. This rendered the
concept meaningless in its loosest interpretation, since 'everybody else'
tended to mean anyone who happened to be talking in a committee at the
time. However, it could just as easily have been the isolated elderly person
for whom an important friend is the television (Taylor and Mullan, 1986).
Nevertheless, the domestic and neighbourhood experience of professional
carers tended to be taken as the (desirable) norm. If 'everybody else' was
taken to be a middle-class member of the caring professions living in a
mortgaged house, this would clearly have little relevance to the experience
of most long-stay hospital residents.

This planning process treatment of normalization only reflected a
national currency in what were termed 'false ideas' by the magazine
Community Living, as described in Table 2.2.

Table 2.2. What is 'normalization'? Reproduced by permission from the
magazine *Community Living* published by 'Good Impressions'

False ideas	Clarification
It means making people 'normal'	It is about value. No one can 'cure' handicaps but people can acquire more appropriate and valued behaviour through services based on positive expectations and proper support

Table 2.2. (*contd*)

False ideas	Clarification
It means treating people as if they were not handicapped or mentally ill … by exposing them to total integration without support. That is a policy of neglect	It does not mean dumping people in the community without specialist help. It provides help where 'devalued people' can mix with ordinary people, not paid to be with them. No argument against paid professional staff, just one in favour of ordinary unremunerated contact as well
It denies people the right to be different — or the opposite — it means that any behaviour, appearance or action is acceptable because free choice and individual differences are 'normal'	It means that services actually encourage people to behave in ways that are valued in our society, which counteracts the devaluating situations in which they mostly find themselves. It does not deny people's right to choose devalued options provided they understand the consequences
It means making it nice for handicapped people. Segregated services are OK if they are like similar services for non-disabled people	It is about creating social change — changing the relationships between those who are devalued and those who are not. It helps increase the physical presence and valued participation of handicapped people in the community. Well-meaning attempts to imitate the real world in segregated settings hinder the achievement of that goal
It is cloud cuckoo land	How can you make progress without some ideal? It is idealistic and compromises have to be made in everyday life
It is common sense	If common sense means ordinary valued living for disabled people then normalization is common sense. But it is very rare and certainly not common
It is anti-professional	Nonsense. It requires highly trained professional staff to support people in ordinary services. There can be a professionalism that does not thrive on increasing social distance

Two perspectives on the planning debates with respect to normalization might be introduced here. Firstly, the idea of the normal experience as a central element of community living can be seen to have its parallel in the original embourgeoisement thesis in sociology: the closer the blue-collar client approaches to bourgeois lifestyle then the more s/he will acquire bourgeois traits of character and habits of mind. This is not far from the ideals of the asylum founders such as Tuke and Pinel. They felt that to treat patients as they would their own dinner party guests would be a core element in restoring a sense of well-being. That asylums quickly became full up despite these efforts, and that blue-collar workers did not become middle class, should warn us of the problems associated with prescribing normal activities for people with mental illness. Where the normal is taken for granted, and where the normal activities that are desirable are believed to be culturally shared or common ones, it is difficult to make any connection with normalization programmes (Jones, Tomlinson and Anderson, 1991).

These comments highlight the irrelevance of normalization if it is conceived only as doing 'normal' things and taking part in 'normal' activities. This defect, or flexibility, in the interpretation of normalization made it open to ridicule among medical and nursing staff, who tended to take up Furlong's position outlined above, that the 1980s asylum population consisted mainly of a hard core of largely intractable patients who would be very difficult to engage in 'normal-seemingness'. So, for example, where the would-be normalizers put forward a scheme for residents of a proposed hostel to be supported in taking up small-scale horticulture in the large garden, since this was what everybody else liked to do, the opponents argued that patient participation in such activity was a completely unrealistic and naive idea. In one sense clearly it was. Patients themselves had not spontaneously shown interest in such a scheme and it did not arise from any exploration of the kind of things that they liked doing or some personal skill that they might be interested in developing. However, in another it provided an opportunity that would be needed, among many others, were any improvement in quality of life to be available to patients coming out of hospital.

Normalization in living accommodation

The most extensive discussions on 'normalization' principles in the vulgarized terms already outlined took place in the project teams that were set up to work out the architectural design of the new community units. These teams were composed of the care professions, planners, managers, architects and building works staff. In their meetings, many members made conscientious efforts to keep to what they regarded as core normalization principles. For example, one team debated whether there should be separate entrances to each of two floors of a building that was to house 16 elderly people. With each floor comprising a self-contained unit for eight, the debate was about whether to have doorways opening separately to each set of rooms or whether to have a common entrance. Since it was common for flats to have shared entrance halls with one another, it was decided that a shared entrance could be justified. Another project team realized that fish knives and forks had been included in the order of cutlery. 'I don't have fish knives and forks in my home,' commented the architect, 'does anybody really have fish knives and forks these days?' Thus normalization had become an architectural design principle before it had been adopted as a rehabilitation philosophy from which design might later follow. A community living questionnaire similar to that used by the Polytechnic of Central London is shown in Figure 2.1.

In a study of community carried out by the author and students at the Polytechnic of Central London, people's subjective sense of there being a community in their area was found to vary according to what social activities they pursued within it. Carry out the following exercise to evaluate your own sense of community.

1. Form into groups of four or five.

2. Each member of the group answer the questionnaire below, relating it to your own home circumstances.

3. Share your results with other members of the group.

4. Consider the implications of this for the integration into communities of the long-stay residents of mental hospitals.

Questionnaire

1. Do you ever go anywhere with neighbours?
   (such as to the shops, post office, vets etc.)   YES/NO

   Please specify ....

   If your answer is Yes, are these trips generally a result of chance meetings or are they planned in advance?
   ....

2. Do you ever take part in any social activities with neighbours? (this can include anything from a Queens Jubilee type street party to meeting in a pub)   YES/NO

   Please specify ....

   If your answer is Yes, are these activities generally a result of chance meeting or are they planned in advance?
   ....

3. Do you feel that you belong to this (i.e. your home) area in any sense? If so, how?
                                                                            YES/NO

   Please specify ....

4. Do you consider that there is a community in this (your home) area?   YES/NO

   If YES, what features do you think best describe the community?
   ....

   If NO, why do you think this is?
   ....

Figure 2.1 Questionnaire adapted from the original one used in the Polytechnic of Central London 1991 study.

Nevertheless, there were some projects in which staff did seek to follow the authentic normalization tenets more closely and wished to avoid making choices on behalf of patients. Those developing such projects immediately became the primary antagonists for the medical and nursing staff, who saw such goals as fantasy. It was around these projects that the major flashpoints in the closure process were to occur, principally because the conflicts of principle underlying them had not received a considered airing in the planning process.

INTERPROFESSIONAL AND INTER-AGENCY CONFLICTS

When the NETRHA closures programme was decided upon it was immensely controversial, as I have discussed elsewhere (Tomlinson, 1991). Looking back, the Regional Treasurer, who had played a key role in the decision making, drew particular attention to the fact that there were conflicts both within professions and between them.

What were the conflicts about?

Psychiatrists

Psychiatrists were the least divided group, the majority arguing that it was necessary both to develop community services and to retain the asylums. The sporting analogy of the asylums as 'back-stops' was often used to describe their role. The psychiatrists distrusted the motives of the Regional Health Authority and believed that no change that involved a decision about closure before new services had been established could be a change for the good. The question of whether new services in the community could do the job as well as those in the large hospitals had to be resolved first. Whatever calculations were produced by NETRHA, the old story of mental hospital physicians being treated as barefoot doctors who could not be trusted to get patients out into the community themselves, was being played out. As psychiatrists were low in the ranks of medicine, the RHA was treating their advice in a cavalier fashion.

A major concern of psychiatrists was that the role of the asylums was being misrepresented. District General Hospital beds could not take over their function. Neither would non-nursing staff in community projects be able to tolerate the antisocial or asocial behaviour of many long-term asylum residents. On the one hand, such residents would almost certainly be rejected by the managers of community facilities because of an ingrained lack of social discipline and insight. On the other hand, caring for such residents would not be a rewarding task for enthusiastic community workers. This was because they would find their clients fundamentally unresponsive and uncommunicative, and it was likely that they would remain so despite the improvement in their environment outside hospital. Removing the back-stop would also leave the housing needs of chronic mentally ill people at the mercy of local authorities. The local authorities were not known to have given any particular priority to this client group in the past.

Notwithstanding, a minority group among the psychiatrists favoured abandoning the asylums. Some of them took the radical position of insisting that all future services should be based within the boundaries of the district in which patients were ordinarily resident. However, others, whom Bromley (1984) calls the 'hesitant supporters', considered that there ought to be, in addition, some 'specialist' units provided on an asylum-type site located to serve several districts. As already noted, NETRHA had implicitly accepted the validity of this argument by opting for only partial closure at Friern. The rationale for 'specialist services' on a 'mini mental hospital' scale was two-fold. Firstly, the services would draw on relatively rare expertise offered within the mental hospitals for the rehabilitation of those extremely withdrawn and unco-operative patients who did not benefit from the DGH regimes. Secondly, there were small groups of patients such as those suffering mental illness as a result of brain damage, who were not sufficiently numerous in any one district to warrant special attention but who, in a mental hospital catchment of half a million people, did constitute 'material' for a specialty.

Nursing staff

At operational levels, nursing staff tended to leave the centre of the debate to psychiatrists, administrators and treasurers, and it was only in a few cases that they played a major planning role. Bromley again points out that, as psychiatric nurses (rather than as general nurses) they lacked proper representation on planning bodies. By 1985, the Griffiths reorganization was to further undermine their position. The irony of this local situation was that, at Regional Health Authority level, it was nursing officers who were the leaders of change.

Nevertheless, at Friern and Claybury, it was the nursing staff who made the first broad estimates of the level of care which their in-patient population would require in the future. As one might expect, they predicted that the majority would require nursing care. If the nurses' views were accepted, then on the face of it, the closure would provide considerable opportunities for career advancement. However, the key issue for nurses was the question of their own 'reprovision' and they were not given the 'no-redundancy' guarantee that their trade union representatives required. Nursing staff in Friern and Claybury were mostly against closure, but they were not in a good position to advance their case. So far as issues concerning philosophy of care were concerned, nursing staff were in a difficult position. On the one hand, they wanted nursing skills and care to be recognized, and for regimes of a like kind to be implemented in the community; on the other, they tended to argue that the resident patient

population in the 1980s had not responded to their best efforts at rehabilitation. What justification was there, then, for nursing care to be axiomatic
in the community rather than any other form of skilled care? This was the
fundamental difficulty in arguing for recognition to be given to nursing
skills in the future care of the long-stay residents.

In 1987, a University Health Services Group was commissioned to work
at Claybury Hospital on a staff development programme (Health Care
Research Associates, 1987). In a series of group interviews that involved
most of the staff, the researchers began by asking them the question 'What
is reprovision?' They found responses to this question to be largely
negative. The responses fell into three categories. The first the researchers
labelled 'don't know and denial', since it was 'not unusual for the question
to be met by blank looks and silence'. The second class of response consisted of factual definitions, such as 'It will be a better life for patients, a
more realistic life'. However, 'by far the most common response to the
question, "What is re-provision?" was a strong and frequently emotional
statement about its negative effects'. This was the third class of response
and perhaps can be summed up best by the phrase 'It's a taking away' used
by one respondent to describe what was interpreted as the taking away of
jobs and of the rehabilitation of patients.

In part, the rejection of reprovision stems from the fact that the retention
of any residual hospital services at Claybury had been ruled out by
Regional and District planners. Negative attitudes tended to be seen as a
kind of inevitable fighting against the dying of the light. Yet at Banstead,
the first large hospital serving London to close in 1986, the argument of
staff that long-stay patients would be best served by continued institutional
care was accepted. Indeed, it became the basic argument to justify the
transfer of patients to an adjacent upgraded hospital (Kensington and
Chelsea AHA, 1979).

The reservations of nursing staff about closure. As a founder member of TAPS,
my own 'observer-as-participant' role has been to monitor and evaluate
how decisions on different models of community services have been implemented. In the course of attending more than 400 planning meetings, I
found the following concerns about community care to be prevalent among
nursing staff:

1. There was great scepticism about the 'normalization' approaches, which
   focus on chronic patients achieving higher levels of 'functioning' in, for
   example, communication skills. For many of this group, hospital staff
   would have lived through several attempts at rehabilitation, only to see
   hopes dashed by the inadequate coping of the patients when discharged
   into the community. Even the communal and semi-supervised living
   arrangements of group homes and hostels have proved inadequate to
   support most chronic patients. Typically, so the argument runs, a resident's thoughts and behaviour will have become more deluded and

bizarre at the same time as s/he has chosen to stop taking medication. The resident may become unduly suspicious of, or aggressive towards the others in the home. When fellow residents' own tolerance levels are not particularly high, tensions soon rise. Then, in keeping with the pattern of previous years, the 'problem resident' will be re-admitted to hospital to be stabilized again before the next period of 'community remission'. Breaking this pattern has been beyond the best efforts of hospital staff. How then, asked many nursing staff, could the idealists, who believed that dependent behaviour stemmed from the rules and sanctions of the institution, possibly be taken seriously?

2. Probably the key issue for nurses in the hospitals was that, in the community, non-nursing staff would not be able to detect fact from fiction in the accounts that patients give of themselves. They would not be able to recognize from withdrawal or ritualistic behaviour the occasions when a client is falling ill, and would leave it too late to intervene. Most dangerously, in their view, non-nursing staff would collude with clients who dislike taking medication and impute harmful effects to it. The net result of such a process would be distress and, in these instances again, re-admission for patients who had been discharged from hospital. They would be subjected once more to being 'medicated from the trolley' and placed under some form of structured regime until their mental state has re-stabilized. Lay people, however caring and well-intentioned, show a lack of ability to recognize all the manifestations of madness. This is a very significant failing. As a consequence, staff of institutions believed that something akin to nursing observation would have to be retained in future services.

3. Hospital staff doubted the wisdom of giving more free choice and more opportunity to patients to devise their own weekly diary of activities. From their own experience of implementing rehabilitation programmes, they believed that close supervision is required to ensure that patients do not go into a process of morbid decline. Without being pushed into undertaking activity that they would not voluntarily have engaged in (e.g. by being kept out of locked dormitories during the day), patients have often tended to withdraw from social interaction, take to their beds, decline to go to workshops, and neglect to change or wash their clothes. Their principal activities might be reduced to those of drinking tea and smoking cigarettes.

Social workers

Social work planners welcomed the closure initiative but had reservations about the funding of it, fearing that responsibility would be off-loaded onto them. In terms of strategy, however, they were as divided as any profession. On the one hand, there were those who regarded closure as an opportunity for filling in gaps in local authority provision of after-care, which had long been 'patchy'. This group tended to feel that social workers' ideological preferences for patient choice, non-restrictive settings, and a non-residential focus of service would have to be reconciled with the prevailing ideology of medical and nursing staff if Social Services departments were to have any roles as service providers. This was pragmatic recognition of the fact that the NHS held the resources for switching to the community.

While all the professions involved were being consulted, it inevitably reflected the corporate dominance within the NHS of medicine and management. Social Services would have to fall into line, and they would have to hope that NHS ideas would be influenced by their own ideas. However, the radical social work wing rejected this strategy because it would mean users of services being saddled with more of the same, if, in the instance of reprovision, with much greater levels of care and supervision. The staple fare would still be the rather traditional forms of adult fostering, short-stay hostels and group homes, which did not give the opportunities for independent non-stigmatized living that many patients were thought to desire. Moreover, compromise would mean that a once-and-for-all chance to shift the service toward domiciliary support and away from in-patient beds would be lost. Conflict between these groups was mostly concealed, although it did break out in social service-only settings. In one moving interview that the author carried out, a Principal Social Worker argued passionately that the whole 'buildings-led' planned retrenchment of the hospitals was totally ignoring the individual needs of residents and was not enabling them to choose their own placement and be supported in activities and employment, and remarked:

> '*I would like to see a labour-intensive and not capital-intensive service. All ideas flow from this initial statement of philosophy — what people do to and with the recovering mentally ill. I wouldn't build a single day centre. A lot of staff, professionals (are needed), not necessarily social workers ... It pains me to see millions of pounds go into specialized apartheid group facilities for this group of people.*'

This team leader had worked at Friern for some years, and the pain that she felt at the spectacle of the planning process unfolding was born partly of despair that her management colleagues in social services would ever understand the needs of the client group. For her, the management team in that particular borough was just colluding with the top-down health authority approach.

Within the radical social work wing were those who followed faithfully, some might say with zeal, authentic normalization principles and attempted to implement them, after the fashion of the 'passing' schema, through reprovision. These advocates managed to obtain Health Authority funding in two specific instances. Although the projects were not proposed by Social Services departments, the departments were their chief supporters, and most of their staff came from backgrounds within the field of social work (for the views of basic-grade social workers in the hospital see Chapter Three).

Administrators

As a group, administrators were torn between following medical advice, which they usually did, and having to carry out a fiat from above, in other words, to make plans for the replacement of the mental hospital. Therefore they looked either to the 'hesitant supporters' among the psychiatrists or, in one or two instances, they sought the advice of District 'Community Physicians', the public medical officers of the Health Authorities who stood in for psychiatrists where the latter were not interested in closure and declined to take part in the planned replacement of the asylums. The pressure on administrators tended perhaps to draw out their innate conservatism. While they were going ahead, with misgivings and at the risk of some rejection from those with whom they had collaborated in consensus management, they would want to ensure that any proposals would not be considered too outlandish by non-participant colleagues (the 'rump psychiatrists').

How were the conflicts handled?

The conflicts were handled through a network of committees. These were, in the main, convened formally within the NHS structure with representatives of other bodies invited to participate. This mode of proceeding derived from the fact that it was the NHS that was paying for reprovision. Though there were several attempts by the non-NHS partners to have the issues dealt with through the 'joint consultative' committees (by which statutory and voluntary sectors formally apprised each other of their views and plans), and therefore to have more parity in discussions, decisions were not made through that route.

Within the NHS communication network, administrative culture was predominant and it was a culture that avoided conflict wherever possible. Clashes of principle, for instance between the apologists of mini-asylums and the applied normalization zealots, were rarely articulated. They never took the form of detailed options appraisal of the different model services on offer. The possibility of a formal trial or experimental service in the short term, while longer-range work went on, was not seriously explored. Advocacy of patients' interests was an issue but was not considered material to the big decisions about new types of service, since it would relate to the individual's right to receive advice and to refuse placements offered.

Entrenched positions

Apart from the polarization of views around normalization already discussed, three issues on which relatively entrenched positions emerged were:

1. Whether asylum could be created in the community without the space and physical separation of the large hospital sites;
2. Whether preventive and crisis management teams had any role to play in the care of people with chronic mental illness; and
3. Whether people who had either failed in successive community placements in the past or had been unacceptable to social services and voluntary organizations could ever be placed outside hospitals such as the two to be closed.

NETRHA deliberately did not lay down any guidelines as to how these issues might be resolved. Each District Health Authority was encouraged to come up with its own philosophy in collaboration with local authorities and voluntary groups. Nevertheless, NETRHA offered advice when it was sought. Specimen architectural designs for long-stay residential accommodation and 'standard operational policies' for such facilities were produced as models, but in no sense were these intended for slavish adoption. These model designs were, however, clearly important for District Planners lacking, like most of those involved in this area of NHS activity, experience with which to develop the solutions. NETRHA architects were suggesting 24-place nursing homes as long-stay residential accommodation and for district officers without the time or planning structure to look beyond off-the-shelf designs, such models were to be of considerable help. It remained a task for the District Authorities to choose between the models of care tentatively offered by the NETRHA and others they might discover (such as those with a non-residential peripatetic staff bias), or to find a compromise between them. From an administrative point of view, that process of choosing was difficult for DHAs.

Rather than explicitly choosing one model in preference to another, the Health Authorities 'froze' the philosophical differences underpinning rival models within their development plans. They achieved this by adopting both a cautious solution, in the form of residential care homes with day care on site, and an adventurous solution, in the form of the outreach care offered by the Community Mental Health centres. This enabled the authorities to adopt a regional health authority plan for an intensively staffed 24-place nursing home for long-stay patients and, at the same time, to propose a totally different service model through which the same client group could be supported by Community Mental Health Centres. There was thus an obvious and acknowledged conflict between the two models of care being built into the implementation process. Very reasonably, therefore, planners adopted the principle of 'flexibility' in the evolution of services: information on the successes and failures of the schemes that opened in the early stages of the reprovision process was intended to be used to adjust those projects that were scheduled for later implementation. However, with that principle adopted, the unresolved conflicts of participants were carried forward into the process of architectural design and commissioning of works.

Whatever its attractions, it is not clear to what extent the principle of flexibility was ever a realistic organizing concept, given the lengthy planning and design cycles for capital projects in both the NHS and Local Government. The more planning progressed, the less flexibility in implementation remained. Moreover, the vested interests of professional groups in projects increased at each stage.

It was clearly difficult to draw up design specifications for the Community Mental Health Centres, given the uncertainties of the care professions about how they would operate. If residential and nursing care requirements were dealt with elsewhere, their role was incipiently a peripheral one. It was, in any case, much easier for planning and design staff to build hospitals, or at least recognizable medical and nursing establishments. Participants felt more comfortable with the self-contained residential and day-care pattern of service. As the planning debate receded and the specifics of site purchase, architecture, and recruitment advanced, the Community Mental Health Centres tended to be seen as making a supplementary contribution to the reprovision task in hand. As one person put it, they were the icing on the cake.

Administrative culture

Practical issues, such as the requirement for detail in lengthy cycles of project development, eroded the planners' vision of flexibility. However, more abstract issues were also relevant — in particular the very nature of NHS decision-making. Hunter (1980) characterized the process of change in the NHS as 'guided incrementalism', where the smallest change to an existing policy is favoured. Glennerster and his colleagues (1982) described their own study of policy-making in the NHS in terms of 'administrative anthropology', in which bureaucracy has rules, customs and myths particular to it. Drawing on my own and others' observations, four keys elements in this 'administrative culture' that are directly related to decision-making for reprovision emerge:

1. Value clashes are side-stepped. Obvious philosophical differences, such as those between the 'public health' and 'protective care' models, are acknowledged by participants as a matter of course. However, when it is clear that there is no ready solution to the conflict, it is either left to be resolved as detailed project work unfolds, or discussed in an *ad hoc* way in the round of informal and chance meetings that take place outside the closure planning committees.
2. Public dispute is avoided. Representatives of the same group do not dispute each other's view in a multi-group discussion. Such dispute would threaten 'in-group' or corporate loyalties.

3. Discussions of conflict are not allowed to reach a climax. There is a shared assumption in the British administrative setting that 'live' working through of conflict is usually non-productive. This is often given as a reason to 'take this issue outside the meeting'. In part, this stems from the convention that professionals hold each other in mutual regard. Working through conflict threatens that comfortable convention.
4. Participants are depersonalized. Opinions are not things that are owned by individuals. Discussions commonly begin with the statement that 'there is a view that such and such..' and then that 'the contrary view is something else ...'.

In summary, the resolution of sensitive conflict is avoided in principle. Hence the testing of different care philosophies against each other is contrary to the administrative culture. Flexibility about the options for service reprovision provided an apparent means of resolving the conflict between competing models of care, but did not offer a way of resolving the conflicts within the administrative culture.

Handling conflicts

Billig and his colleagues (1988) have carried out research into what they call 'ideological dilemmas' in decision-making. One of their concerns has been with the processes by which conflicts are handled in multidisciplinary team-working. They discuss four assumptions of inter-professional decision-making which, taken together, provide an instructive parallel to the features of administrative culture described in this section. The assumptions are that:

1. As a result of a common foundation in science, the technical knowledge of any one professional discipline is equal in value to the technical knowledge of any other.
2. A multidisciplinary approach to the problems presented by clients involves pooling of knowledge and recognition of the limitations of each discipline. The attitude of any one contributor should be 'I've reached the limit of my knowledge and I hand it over to you'. Then a consensus emerges from the pooled technical views.
3. An ethos of democratic, co-operative sharing of tasks is, paradoxically, necessary to preserve the authority and status by which each profession is accorded a ranking. A 'politeness maxim' is invoked by which high-status professional groups invite those in lower-status groups to contribute or take the lead on certain tasks, rather than to order them to do things and ruin the ethos of democracy that is necessary for harmonious working. Underlying this ethos are the principles of liberalism and anti-authoritarianism of the wider society.
4. The person of the expert is differentiated from the expert's knowledge.

The last point is very close to my own observation about the de-personalizing of conflict, but it is the third point that I feel picks up on a key feature of administrative culture and decision-making.

Billig *et al.* (1988) cite Middleton and Mackinlay's 1987 discussion of an interaction between a higher- and a lower-ranking professional to make the point clear. The lower-ranking professional, a nursery nurse, explains to the researchers that the multidisciplinary team in which she works genuinely functions as a group of equals: 'We all do everybody else's job and we all take advice from each other'. However, when a higher-ranking speech therapist from the team enters the room where this conversation is taking place this image is shattered. The therapist politely asks 'Excuse me, have we got any medicine cups?' She is told by the nursery nurse that there might be some in the drugs cupboard but that the pharmacy stores provide them. This response, Billig suggests, was not what the opening gambit of the speech therapist had sought. The latter then states 'I want it now though' and the nursery nurse obediently responds by searching for the cup.

With the democracy of equals less certain, the speech therapist has to deny that she has in any way invoked her authority over the nursery nurse. She parodies her own phrase 'I want it now' in a humorous tone. In so doing, Billig argues, 'she distances her own command from the sort of authoritarian, military command that would have been unacceptable.'

Blurring of roles

David Billis, an analyst of organizational processes, conceives of the blurring of roles in voluntary organizations between management committees and the paid workers they employ in terms of overlapping circles (Fig. 2.2):

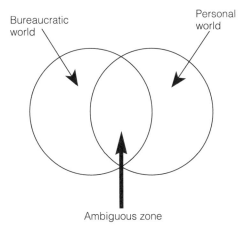

Figure 2.2   Billis' 1984 view of the blurring of the roles in voluntary organizations.

The diagram indicates that in the case of many enthusiasts in the voluntary sector, whether management-committee or paid-employee members, who join for moral and altruistic reasons, their work roles are blurred by definition. Depersonalizing is much more difficult and, in a sense, is not accepted in the voluntary sector culture. Alternatively, arising from the tradition of voluntary Social Work and of Hospital Almoners, the 'official distributors of alms', there is also a blurring of roles in the statutory sector.

Drawing the threads of this discussion together, when we think of innovation in the NHS and the radical change represented by devolution from mental hospitals, it is taking place within a framework of:

1. Democratic pooling of knowledge between the professional groups who are party to decision-making;
2. A hierarchy of professional status that conventionally has to be denied in decision-making in order for the higher orders to elicit the unforced co-operation of the lower orders;
3. Decision-making through consideration of depersonalized proposals. The presenter of these proposals should betray no personal passion but convey only the arguments that can be based on scientific, technical know-how.

In this situation, radical change can occur in one of two ways. It can occur as a result of a paradigmatic shift in the scientific and technical knowledge, in other words a Copernican revolution. Alternatively, it can occur when the high-status professional groups invite others within the decision-making process to introduce new techniques. In mental health, the consultant psychiatrists would be such a group. In NETRHA, managers and planners were not advocating specific project solutions, but at the same time only a small minority of psychiatrists (Bromley's hesitant supporters of reprovision) were acting to facilitate the change.

Product champions

So it is apparent that, within the administrative culture observed by the author, more opportunistic and uneven methods of introducing radical community projects to replace hospital-like care would tend to be prevalent. Stocking's work (1985) suggests for instance that 'product champions' who enjoy high status in their own profession and the respect of colleagues outside their profession might be the bearers of community initiatives. However, as the very term 'product champions' suggests, such advocates of innovations would clearly have made a strong personal commitment to the way of working that they would be seeking to implement. Their passion would be a handicap to acceptance of their proposals. For the correct presentation of proposals in administrative culture, this personal element has to be exorcized. Moreover, product champions, as charismatic leaders, are in any case thin on the ground.

The introduction of radical changes as a result of external manipulation, such as through command from the top (RHA) or through public pressure, was not in evidence where Friern and Claybury were concerned.

The Grove: a case study of the administrative process

The Grove was one of the first resettlement facilities planned as part of the closure of Friern and Claybury hospitals and was to take patients from both hospitals. The Grove is a detached residence dating from the Queen Anne period and belonging to the local Council, and which had by the 1980s fallen into a state of some disrepair.

Early stages. The early stages of the planning process for the DHA that was concerned in this property were ones in which 'sites were looking for client groups' as the District Planning Officer put it. On the one hand, his officers were in difficulties without the advice of the psychiatrists since, in this district, they had not been able to agree with the proposition that closure was feasible or desirable. Both the senior Social Service staff and senior Health Authority staff felt this lack of engagement as a significant loss. On the other hand, this DHA had also been awarded the biggest task of the programme, to create over 400 reprovision places within the district. The priority attached to finding sites was wholly understandable in these circumstances. The DHA had adopted an initially cautious reprovision plan, which envisaged most long-stay and elderly patients being trans-ferred to community nursing homes and hostels. Only a minority of them, it was felt, would be able to be resettled in more independent accom-modation. Clearly, many sites would be needed for these facilities, although some would be situated at the General Hospital site.

The Grove Hospital was seized on as a building that could provide residential and day care for the minority from Friern and Claybury who could benefit from the traditional Social Services/voluntary sector after-care. The DHA would pay for the refurbishment of the building and for Social Services to manage and staff a rehabilitation scheme on the site. So far so good. For the less malleable majority of the long-stay hospital, several different projects were being proposed. At one end of the spectrum was a rehabilitation settlement of 50 places, to be run after Wing and Furlong's (1986) 'haven' principles, on a hospital site. At the bottom of the stairway would be highly staffed houses, with residents attending on-site day hospital care. As their rehabilitation progressed they would move up the Haven site stairway to less highly staffed houses and hopefully, at the top, move to sheltered employment and into supported hostels.

The other end of the rehabilitation spectrum proposed in this district was represented by adult fostering, and small staffed group homes in 'ordinary houses in ordinary streets'. The planning philosophy evolved toward one of 'core and cluster' to underpin this range. 'Core and cluster' was an estab-lished principle in the field of learning difficulties and it was the Nursing

Officer most involved in planning who felt it had a useful application to the mental health field. Basically, the NHS would run the 'core' facilities such as the Haven complex, for the more dependent patients, while the Social Services and voluntary sector would run the cluster facilities for the less dependent minority group of patients. The Grove and several staffed group homes to be scattered across the district would make up cluster residences.

Although this arrangement was administratively easy to grasp, several problems of application and interpretation quickly arose with the core and cluster concept. Core and cluster was useful as an organizing concept because it masked several unresolved disputes such as who would control the assessment and selection process — would it be the consultant psychiatrists? Who would attend to preparation of patients for community living? What criteria would apply to distinguish core from cluster residents? Would nurses 'assist' in (social work) cluster teams? Would social workers 'assist' in core (NHS) teams, where follow-up of clients between facilities was desirable? It was also clear that there was an unstated element of competition between the Haven, which was situated right at the western end of the district, and the Grove at the eastern end. The Haven was an NHS nursing facility that appeared to encompass both core and cluster functions all on one site, while the Grove would be operating as an independent unit that was not planned to be operationally associated with a core unit.

Support for the project. The two key backers of the Grove project in the planning team were a Social Services Manager and the DHAs District Medical Officer. They ensured that the project was placed firmly in the DHA reprovision funding plan. However, they were not clinical product champions. So when the project was transferred across from the planning team to the DHA's Estates Development staff, in order for building works specifications and contracting work to be done, it spent a lonely, long and unchampioned time being assessed for its feasibility on these criteria. Building costs inflation continued to escalate, while predicted staffing costs already looked on the high side. The unresolved clinical issues that it carried only made matters worse.

By this stage, a new General Manager had dispensed with the untenable core-and-cluster concept, redesignating the Grove and the Haven as both belonging to the category of 'intensive rehabilitation' facilities. Of course this only served to make the Grove more jealously regarded as a competitor to DHA rehabilitation — especially when the DHA's own projects were not so well-advanced within the planning and development system. The building works criteria had begun to undermine the feasibility of the Grove with several complicated legal and contracting issues frustrating the Director of Social Services. At the same time, the District General Manager became increasingly concerned at the cost of the project, in both revenue and capital terms. After many delays, and angry exchanges over them between members of the Council and the Regional and District Health Authorities, the DHA finally agreed to restorative work commencing at the Grove.

The opening of the project. When the project opened, with the Manager being (ironically, in view of the competition between agencies over who was doing the rehabilitation work in reprovision) a nurse from a mental hospital by background, it won some acclaim. It was even subjected to a 'good practices' feature in one of the trade magazines. All the first group of residents were resettled from the Grove to more independent accommodation. However, after this early period, the supply of residents from the mental hospitals began to dry up, largely because of the unresolved issues about who was in control of the selection procedure and who was carrying out rehabilitation. At the time of writing, the project could be considered expensive because it operated with what were effectively 40% voids. At the same time, a crisis in capital funding slowed the reprovision programme at Claybury, thus adding further to the difficulties of the Grove in its operation from that hospital.

Administrative culture. This short history of the Grove thus exhibits all the features of a planning process in which administrative culture is dominant:

1. Flexibility as an organizing principle, in this instance with the core-and-cluster approach providing a conceptual shroud;
2. Unworked-through value disputes over the professional control and technical management of assessment, selection, resettlement and rehabilitation;
3. A lack of product champions, with projects being proposed on political and availability of buildings-led criteria;
4. Cost-effectiveness issues of building and contracting work becoming predominant by default;
5. The success, in the project's terms, of its staff resettling all the original complement of residents that moved in to the Queen Anne mansion, being devalued. This was the more notable given the psychiatrists' predictions that patients who could benefit from social services after-care had long since left Friern and Claybury by the time reprovision arrived as an initiative; and
6. Comparative evaluation of differing forms of care becoming increasingly difficult.

The fact that the project achieved some success despite this developmental background is probably mostly attributable to the efforts of the staff appointed to run it. Inevitably, their work has been undermined because of the re-emergence of the unresolved issues that were cast off in the implementation process after the adoption of the organizing principle of flexibility.

The committee behaviour underlying reprovision planning as a whole cannot be discussed in detail here, but its existence meant that the major issues were not worked through in any systematic way. This was partly because participants paid 'lip-service' to the convention that all the professions involved were of equal standing in relation to each other. The hierarchy of status, as Billig's work shows, could not be invoked. Was it rehabilitation that was to be carried out with long-stay patients (a largely lapsed medical and nursing staff role) or was it long-term social support (an as yet barely extant social work role)? Here was a most uncomfortable conflict, which if explored would obviously threaten the convention of professional equality. This avowed blindness to professional background operated in a similar way to colour blindness in a multi-racial society. There was the same outcome, that professions that had the greatest power, authority and status, whether their representatives were reacting to proposals or making them, exerted the greatest influence in shaping the new services.

Implications for future practice

Conflicts about the role of mental hospitals themselves, the possibility of rehabilitation for their long-stay residents and about philosophies of rehabilitation were not resolved, but were shelved within administrative culture. Thus there was a tendency for the 'least disruptive' alternatives to mental hospitals to be adopted, with a focus on grouping patients according to their assessed dependency or disability. In turn, the focus on staff specialties in responding to these dependencies and disabilities meant that buildings to house established practices in the specialties came to be a focus for planning effort. The untried and untested processes of enabling asocial non-communicative, long-stay patients to make choices and of finding them residences not daubed with the 'mental health' label were very much at the margins and extremes. They were accepted by most participants as perhaps desirable in principle, but only in the future and thus not feasible within reprovision. It was a case of small steps rather than a giant leap for mankind, as one Regional nursing officer put it. This meant that users' views were considered very late in the day and the models of service that 'went out to public consultation', as administrators put it, could hardly be considered popular. They had been derived 90% from the drift of professional conflicts toward a position of least change in terms of philosophies of care. The drift took place within the administrative culture. If this situation is to be avoided in future, then debates in that culture will have to be broadened outward from the professional providers of services toward the public and consumers.

It may be countered immediately that if the public and many long-stay residents had their way the asylums would stay, but clearly the goal is consumer choice between a range of possibilities rather than asylum or non-asylum places. Public consultation was an initial feature of NETRHA policy making. Perhaps an element of popular choice between available models of care could also be introduced.

It is true that, in general, public interest in community psychiatric care has been limited, but in areas with active voluntary mental health groups (e.g. local branches of MIND) much more public discussion has taken place. This suggests that direct public involvement in defining care requirements may be possible in some districts. Also, community development workers employed by local authorities liaise extensively with generic community groups not organized around mental health; they have a detailed know-ledge of specific local concerns for those suffering mental illnesses. In some areas, they have facilitated the growth of support groups among carers and relatives of people with mental illness, and befriending schemes with the participation of people from the neighbourhood. The experience of these workers should be made available to planners. Furthermore, direct contact with the users of mental health services has increased among NHS managers in the last few years. Some user groups have had modest success in changing intentions so that plans move more towards providing the types of facilities they want.

If professionals cannot, in concert, decide on the most effective service, at the least models of service that are desired locally can be evolved. Moreover, broadening the debate may alter professional attitudes. Relevant issues can easily be put to one side in the administrative culture. Outside it, participants will have little compunction about raising and addressing them. In such a context, more informed decisions can be made.

Future staff involvement

On the basis of the progress of those patients who have currently been resettled in the community, the welfare of Friern and Claybury leavers seems assured. More than 400 have been followed up and asked whether they prefer community living to hospital living, as well as being assessed on clinical criteria: they overwhelmingly prefer their community placements.

One could conclude that nursing staff are not needed in community placements, since patients have left hospital in the first wave of reprovision to as many new non-nursing regimes as to nursing facilities, but this is to run ahead of the process. Only a part of the range of the types of nursing care given in the asylums has yet been provided in the community. The more dependent and disturbed patients have yet to move.

It was noted earlier that in a few projects normalization principles were followed rigorously. The TAPS findings seem to suggest that the high expectations of normalization and of patients attaining greater levels of competence and self care have not been borne out. A member of staff at one of the projects commented:

'There's now an acknowledgement that these are very dependent individuals who need physical care. We've got an overqualified staff team who are not there for bum wiping or for opening a can of beans... Long-term care is needed but we can still fulfil values and options... But we're not there to cure people and we're not there to turn people into middle-class people choosing this, that and the other'.

Clearly hospital staff are not going to warm to planning for the reprovision of their wards unless they are truly participants in the process, and asked for their preferred options for new community services, rather than being consulted after pre-emptive planning team decisions. The creation of new forms of care can only benefit from full assessment of the advantages and disadvantages of the old ones.

The author's experience as a carer in different hospitals is an additional means of gaining insight to the research reported in this chapter. The author is the first to be aware of, and to warn against, the creation of 'wards in the community'. However, a dialogue that begins from 'grass roots' patient and staff perspectives on the one hand, and planners' wider community care goals on the other, will widen the span of feasible approaches to reprovision and give consultation a higher rating in the process.

Conclusion

What stands out from this discussion of the rundown of these two hospitals is that a straightforward transfer of care from hospital to community is taking place. Finally, after many years of public concern about the conditions of the asylums, their residents are being moved to placements in the catchment areas, which provide a vastly improved standard of accommodation and amenities, and a much increased ratio of staff to patients. Clinicians who have followed up the progress of the 400 long-stay patients who have moved so far have concluded that: (a) movers much prefer their community settings to hospitals; and (b) their mental state remains stable after resettlement. It is difficult to argue with the judgement that, so far, this community care programme is working well.

Mental hospitals are an administrative anachronism and managers have needed to reorganize them in such a way that they can be dispersed and repackaged as local, or as district, or as community units. How this was to be done was a task they passed on to the caring professions. A clear-cut corporate professional project, possibly 'a patriarchal professional project' therefore emerged (Witz, 1990). Male-dominated professions such as psychiatry, psychiatric nursing, and health administration attempted to develop technical knowledge-based responses to the requirements of closure. Patients were consigned to chronicity in the community without their proper involvement in decision-making or anything approaching partnership between consumers and the state. Although it must be acknowledged that gaining such involvement is a goal that is very difficult to achieve for managers in mental health, the weight of the prescriptive judgements of professional carers about specific medical and nursing care regimes required in the community was all too striking. Five key elements in policy making contributed to this outcome:

1. The need for community services being equated with the need for new buildings to replace those of the hospital;
2. Non-recognition of the experience of the enthusiasts for resettlement among nursing staff in the asylums, and thus failure to engage their concerns and interests in a planning partnership;
3. Administrative culture preventing the working through of conflicts in care philosophy and, as a corollary, devaluing of input from the marginalized lower-ranking professions such as social work; and
4. Underestimation of the potential for patients and relatives to be involved in determining the future pattern of services. For the moment, this process has left all the major issues for mental health services in the 21st century untouched.

REFERENCES

Barclay, P. (1982) *Social Workers: Their Role and Tasks*. Bedford Square Press. London.

Billig, M., Condor, S., Edwards, D., Gane, M., Middleton, D. and Radley, A. (1988) *Ideological Dilemmas*. Sage, London.

Billis, D. *Policy Implementation in the Non-profit Sector*, Undated, unpublished paper, London School of Economics.

Bromley, G. L. (1984) *Hospital Closure: Death of Institutional Psychiatry?* MA Thesis, University of Essex.

Cumberlege, J. (1988) *Neighbourhood Nursing: The focus on care*, Department of Health and Social Security, HMSO, London.

DHSS (1975) *Better Services for the Mentally Ill*. HMSO, London.

Fagin, L. (1985) De-institutionalization. *Bulletin of the Royal College of Psychiatrists*, **9**, 11–12.

Furlong, R. C. S. (1985) Closure of Large Mental Hospitals — Practicable or Desirable?, *Bulletin of the Royal College of Psychiatrists*, **9**, 12–13.

Garelick, A. (1988) The Decision to Close an Area Mental Hospital. *Bulletin of the Royal College of Psychiatrists*, **12**, 15–17.

Glennerster, H., Korman, N., Marslen Wilson, F. and Meredith B. (1982) *Social Planning*. London School of Economics, London.

Hunter, D. J. (1980) *Coping with Uncertainty*. John Riley, Letchworth.

Health Care Research Associates (1987) *Staff and Reprovision: An Assessment of Claybury Hospital*. University of Surrey, Guildford.

Jones, D., Tomlinson, D. R. and Anderson, J. (1991) Asylums and Community Care: plus ça change. *Journal of the Royal Society of Medicine*, **84**, 252–54.

Kensington and Chelsea Area Health Authority (1979) *Report of the Area Psychiatric Services Working Party to the September meeting of the Authority*.

Martin, D. V. (1955) Institutionalization. *Lancet*, **3**, 1188.

Martin, D. V. (1968) *Adventure in Psychiatry*. Cassirer, Oxford.

McKee, L. and Pettigrew, A. (1988) Managing major change, *Health Service Journal*, **98**, 5127, 1358–60.

North East Thames Regional Health Authority (NETRHA) (1983) *Report to the Regional Health Authority on Feasibility Studies on Mental Illness Services in the Catchment Areas of Friern and Claybury Hospitals.* NETRHA, London.

Palmer, I. (1985) State theory and statutory authorities: Points of convergence, *Sociology*, **19**, 4, 274–97.

Ramon, S. (1983) Psychiatria democratica: A case study of the Italian community mental health service. *International Journal of Health Services*, **13 (2)**, 311.

Samson, C. J. (1990) *The Privatization of Mental Health: Political and Ideological Influences in Psychiatric Care in the United States and Great Britain, 1979–1989.* Ph D Thesis, University of California, Berkeley.

Stocking, B. (1985) *Initiative and Inertia.* Nuffield Provincial Hospitals Trust, London.

Taylor, L. and Mullan, B. (1986) *Uninvited Guests.* Chatto and Windus, London.

Team for the Assessment of Psychiatric Services (TAPS) (1988) *Preliminary Report on Baseline Data from Friern and Claybury Hospitals.* NETRHA, London.

Tomlinson, D. R. (1988) *The Administrative Process of Claybury and Friern Reprovision.* NETRHA, London.

Tomlinson, D. R. (1991) Utopia, *Community Care and the Retreat from the Asylums.* Open University Press, Milton Keynes.

Towell, D. and Macausland, T. (1988) *Managing Psychiatric Services in Transition: An Overview.* King Edward Hospital Fund for London, London.

Wing, J. K. and Furlong, R. (1986) A haven for the severely disabled within the context of a comprehensive psychiatric community service, *British Journal of Psychiatry*, **149**, 257–69.

Witz, A. (1990) Patriarchy and professions. *Sociology*, **24 (4)**, 675–90.

Part Two
Being at the receiving end of the closure process

'We turned suffering from the mental hospital out onto the streets, and this led the town to discover its own suffering, which was codified in other separate institutions.'

Franco Basaglia, 1979

3

The perspective of professional workers: living with ambiguity, ambivalence and challenge

SHULAMIT RAMON

Apart from one study on three teams of social workers facing the closure of a psychiatric hospital reported at the end of this chapter, there are no studies directly focused on workers' reaction to such closures. We need to understand why this is the case, despite the fact that professionals lead and work in such hospitals, and despite the fact that many psychiatric hospitals have closed down since the 1960s in the USA, Italy, Australia, and more recently in Britain too.

The lack of research focused on the professionals in the closure process relates firstly to the understandable interest in what happens to clients during closure. Secondly, it relates to the dominance of a tradition of research in which variables difficult to quantify are better not studied; professional responses to the closure do not lend themselves easily to quantification. Thirdly, in several countries the process of closure is perceived to be administrative in essence, in which professionals are obedient employees. Within such a perspective all of what is required from them is to follow administrative instructions.

It is my profound disagreement with the latter perspective that has led me to become interested in studying professionals' responses to the closure. Having had the privilege of observing the development of the Italian psychiatric reform in several Italian cities (Ramon, 1983, 1985c, 1989, 1990) I have become convinced of the centrality of professionals to the success or failure of any meaningful attempt to change a mental health system. For me, professionals are employees paid to make autonomous decisions and to use discretion, thus, by definition, enjoying an ambiguous position within the bureaucratic structures in which most professionals are working.

In the absence of research on professionals during hospital closure, I have looked at related evidence, such as: (a) observations and writings about the

North American de-institutionalization policies and processes (Castel *et al.*, 1982; Brown, 1985; Bachrach, 1983; Ramon, 1985b); (b) the Italian psychiatric reform, studies on stress experienced by health and mental health professionals at points of transition (Menzies-Lyth, 1988; Payne, 1987; Carson and Bartlett, 1990; Allen *et al.*, 1990); and (c) the findings from my small-scale study (Ramon, 1990).

The more general framework with which to understand the place of professionals in mental health services and the issues they face regularly has come from the sociology and social psychology of professions (Parry and Parry, 1976). Inevitably, this has been modified by my own understanding of the state-of-the-art.

WHAT IS PROFESSIONALISM ABOUT?

Professionals: legitimacy base and sources of ambiguity and ambivalence

Being a professional implies working in a way that follows from acquired professional knowledge and ethics. Professional associations, training bodies, the government, and the general public assume that **both** components — knowledge and ethics — are necessary for the protection of the client from being abused and for ensuring that the client is receiving the best available intervention. Further, it is assumed that professional knowledge **does** exist and offers an improvement on common sense in terms of understanding what happens to people in specific situations, predicting what is likely to happen to them, and in providing a range of skills and interventions with which to solve a difficulty or improve a given state. This is the basis for the belief in professional expertise, and for the considerable social investment in preparing people for professional activity. It is also the foundation for respecting professionals and providing them with adequate signs of social appreciation, such as reasonable salaries and working conditions, as well as symbolic signs of prestige (e.g. calling people by their professional titles, attributing to some professions a predominantly altruistic motivation).

The ethical aspect of professional work is of equal importance in securing that people in need of resolution of a problem, and hence in a vulnerable and dependent position (at least on a temporary basis), will not be exploited for the self-enhancement of the person who provides them with the forms of solution. Ethical behaviour takes many forms, such as prohibiting sexual relationships with a client, financial exploitation, the disclosure of personal information given in the course of a professional encounter to anyone but other professionals involved in working with the same client, as well as treating the client with due respect even when disapproving of a particular act committed by the client. Conflict may arise between the best use of knowledge and acting in accordance to ethical principles. For example, the use of new drugs on prisoners calls for a very delicate balance between the wish to expand knowledge and risking people's lives, however socially devalued they may be.

To ensure that professionals have the right knowledge and ethical base, training bodies have been established, with complex machinery concerning the validation of training programmes and the screening of applicants coming on professional courses.

This description of professionalism as a benevolent instrument has been criticized from two perspectives. Firstly, it has been argued that it fails to take into account the issue of professional power, both the power of individual professionals over individual clients and the power of professional bodies as gate-keepers to becoming and remaining recognized professional figures, stifling innovation and creativity in the process (Johnson, 1973; Friedson, 1970). In addition, professionals act as agents of social control rather than of care (Castel *et al.*, 1982; Ingleby, 1981).

Secondly, it has been argued that, far from being benevolent, professionalism can have a malevolent effect on both the client and the practising professional. In the book *Disabling Professions* Illich (1968) and others have put forward the case that professionalism militates against self and mutual help, personal initiative, and commonsensical understanding. According to this perspective, professionals dictate to people a particular way of understanding their difficulties, their needs, as well as methods of sorting out these issues. This imposition disempowers ordinary people. Furthermore, in some cases it may have an iatrogenic effect, namely harming people instead of helping them.

The 'semi' professions

Professions are by definition applied disciplines, with professional knowledge being tested by its relevance and usefulness to a set of situations that take place in everyday life.

A further distinction is made in differentiating between 'fully-fledged' and 'semi' professions. According to several writers on professionalism, occupations such as social work, nursing and occupational therapy are only 'semi' professions (Etzioni, 1969; Toren, 1972), whereas psychiatry is a 'fully-fledged' profession. By coining this term they mean to say that the knowledge base of these groups is less unique than that of the main professions, in which medicine is included. For example, Toren (1972) highlights that social-work knowledge is taken from several allied disciplines, such as psychology, social policy and sociology. Toren expresses her doubts as to what is unique to social-work knowledge, arguing that a fully-fledged profession can make a justified claim to knowledge that is only its own. In turn, social-work theorists have argued that it is the way in which knowledge from different sources is blended that makes it unique or not, and furthermore it is the way knowledge is applied that is the hallmark of uniqueness in the case of an applied discipline.

Interestingly, the nub of the debate is around theory, rather than around the uniqueness of the role or practice skills associated with it. Perhaps this focus on theory reflects the emphasis of the researchers on these issues, rather than either those of practising professionals or the recipients of their services. It is debatable whether the distinction between fully-fledged and semi professions is useful, apart from highlighting some of the reasons for the different social standing of different professions, and the historical development of disciplines such as nursing in the shadow of a better known and more detailed 'parental' profession. However, it would be unrealistic to ignore the different developmental path of different professions, and their relative strengths and weaknesses along the dimensions of theory articulation, skills, roles and tasks (Ramon, 1985a; Sheppard, 1991).

A crucial point that, in my view, has been ignored in this ongoing debate on professions and professionalism has been the social mandate given to professionals to take the responsibility for calculated risks in predictions and in interventions (Brearly, 1972). This is apparent in law (finding a person guilty or not is a prime example) not less than in medicine (to operate or not to operate, to give a drug that has considerable negative side-effects or not), or in social work (to remove a person from his home to hospital or not, to remove a child from her natural family or not, to let a frail elderly person stay at home or not). One of the primary justifications for the creation of complex accountability structures in human services is the need to ensure adequate consideration of each aspect involved in reaching decisions related to risk-taking, as well as to provide support for the individual worker or team that has the ultimate responsibility for taking the risk and living with its consequences. Thus I am arguing that not only the client lives with the consequences of professional decisions; workers too live with the outcomes of their decision-making, albeit at a different level.

This social mandate to professions implies that they are not only transmitters and interpreters of professional knowledge and representative of their profession. They are also social agents, entitled to exercise both care and control in the process of performing their professional duties. The duality of being a relatively autonomous professional and a social agent simultaneously is one of the main sources of ambivalence and conflict for professionals.

HEALTH-RELATED PROFESSIONS

All of the above is directly related to professions working in the health field. In addition, we need to take into account the specific motivations, satisfactions, frustrations and dilemmas that these professions face.

People enter health- and illness-related work with more than one motive, including the wish to help people, to restore them to health, to establish individualized helping relationships, to gain social status, to prove their abilities, to gain knowledge about the mysteries of life, to earn money with which to enjoy a pleasing standard of living (Becker, 1967). This set of motivations is invariably met in everyday practice by the following dimensions:

1. Failing to help people and failure to restore them to health even when one has given it all of what one has professionally;
2. Living with suffering and destruction; and
3. Working within a large bureaucracy that militates against individual initiative and individualized relationships.

It is easy to see the numerous occasions of frustration resulting from the mismatch of reasons for engaging in health-related professional activity and these dimensions.

Isabel Menzies-Lyth (1988) has studied a large British general hospital at the request of senior members of the nursing hierarchy to advise how to stop the high rate of student nurses leaving before the completion of training. Although her study was conducted more than 30 years ago, its conclusions have retained their validity. On the basis of interviews and observations of nurses' work, she concluded that the discrepancy between the motivation to be a nurse and what student nurses have been asked to do in their everyday work is the dominant reason for leaving the profession. Furthermore, the more able and mature students were leaving. What student nurses have been asked to perform seems to be influenced by institutional defence mechanisms against the anxiety generated by living with suffering and instances of failure to alleviate suffering and restore people to health. In turn, these mechanisms create a defensive culture, which prevails throughout the institution and which militates against being a good nurse, almost forcing individuals to provide an impersonal service, to the dissatisfaction of both nurses and patients. Table 3.1 lists the defence mechanisms suggested by Menzies-Lyth:

Table 3.1. Typical defence mechanisms developed by student nurses in a general hospital.

- Splitting up the nurse-patient relationship (e.g. performing the same task for many patients, rather than most of the tasks with a small number of patients)
- Depersonalization, categorization and denial of the significance of the individual (e.g. talking about the patient as 'the liver case in No. 17')
- Detachment and denial of feelings (e.g. after being reprimanded for crying on the ward)
- Elimination of decisions by ritual task performance (e.g. rigid rules for bed-making and lifting a patient)
- Reducing the weight of responsibility in decision-making by checks and counterchecks (e.g. ensuring that no decisions, however small, are

Table 3.1.   *(contd)*

---

taken by one person, and endlessly counterchecking them after they have been taken)
- Collusive social redistribution of responsibility and irresponsibility (e.g. defining irresponsibility as becoming emotionally attached to a patient and/or skimping boring tasks, attributing irresponsibility to junior nurses only, denying irresponsibility in oneself while attributing it to others)
- Purposeful obscurity in the formal distribution of responsibilities (e.g. giving and having two different task-lists for the same day; difficulties in finding out who is responsible for what)
- Reducing the impact of responsibility by delegation to superiors (e.g. usually delegation implies from the superiors to those below them in the hierarchy. However, nurses tend to require superiors to take more and more of the responsibility, even in cases such as selecting student nurses with whom intermediate staff would want to work for the next six months)
- Idealization and underestimation of personal developmental possibilities (e.g. 'nurses are born, not made'; lack of individual supervision for student nurses)
- Avoidance of change (e.g. increasing the number of regulations and prescriptions when faced with the difficulty of handling a fluctuating workload)

Adapted from Menzies-Lyth (1988).

You are invited to judge from your own experience whether these mechanisms are part of your everyday work experience. You may find it useful to discuss these examples, and the issues they highlight, with your colleagues, fellow students and/or tutors.

Consider with your colleagues, fellow students and tutor, more helpful responses; what can make it feasible for these to be adopted in everyday practice by most of you. Try one of them out; report back to your team, or class, how it went; what went well, what did not go so well, why, and how it can be improved.

Menzies-Lyth proposes that these mechanisms develop as a way of overcoming not only the anxiety provoked by the presence of suffering but by the guilt and infantile fantasies that this anxiety leads to at the unconscious level. It seems to me that both anxiety and the guilt evoked by the realistic limitations of professional competence and organizational framework in combating disease and ill health are perfectly understandable and normal responses to an abnormal situation, even though they are neither the only possible nor the most helpful reactions. Locating them at the unconscious level is not only difficult to prove but is unhelpful in the attempt to support nurses and to encourage the development of a more productive repertoire of collective (institutional) and individual (professional–personal) responses.

Para-professionals in health-related work

In several activities related to professional duties, such as day centres and residential establishments, we will find workers who have not gone through the socially agreed modes of training and are not qualified professionals. Apart from expediency, shortage of staff or financial resources to pay them adequately, it has been argued that some functions are better or at least equally performed by unqualified staff. This argument has been particularly relevant to the aftermath of the de-institutionalization process, in which long-term residents of hospitals are introduced to ordinary living, or in the projects aimed at enabling people with a disability to remain in the community. The reasoning behind it is the claim that para-professionals are less removed from everyday life than are professionals and would therefore be better equipped to prepare people with disabilities for ordinary living, or to maintain them in the community.

The relationships between qualified and unqualified care staff are not easy to sort out in principle. This is compounded now by the realization that there are common skills required for the revalorization of people who have been institutionalized that cut across professional disciplines and disabilities, such as 'the trick of being ordinary' (Brandon, 1989, 1991). Chapter One and Chapter Four provide examples of the work of this group, and some of the issues mentioned in this section.

In everyday work it is possible to delineate lines of responsibility for each group and to acknowledge the value of both contributions, even though tension and conflict may be underlying themes of these seemingly untroubled arrangements.

MENTAL HEALTH WORKERS AND PROFESSIONS: SOURCES OF AMBIGUITY AND AMBIVALENCE

We need to ask ourselves what of the above is of particular relevance to mental health professionals, and whether there are other issues that require our attention before we turn to the specific issues that hospital closure confronts workers with. Professional work in mental health is both an ancient and a modern phenomenon. Psychic healing has been universally practised from time immemorial, given the universality of suffering mental pain, the wish and need to relieve it and the effects it has on functioning. Healers claimed the possession of unique knowledge, and were given the social mandate to exercise this knowledge, take calculated risks and provide care and control. Their source of knowledge was perceived to be divine, coming from supernatural powers and practised as a **disciplined art** by the healer.

In its modern 'reincarnation', mental health work has been associated primarily with medicine on the one hand and with psychology on the other. While there is considerable disagreement on what constitutes good scientific knowledge in mental health, especially along the dichotomy of medicine *versus* psychology, it is important to note that, in relation to both, the emphasis has been and still is on the **scientific basis** of the knowledge and the practice. Thus the disciplined art component is largely ignored, and any claim to a divine source is clearly rejected. It is relatively easy to understand the rejection of the assumption of divine sources as one of the outcomes of the move away from religion as the main source of knowledge.

Understanding the lack of attention to the disciplined art component is both less clear and more complex in the motivation behind it and in its ramifications for mental health workers. It is in part due to the wish to reinforce the scientific status of mental health knowledge and activity, which is based on the assumption that Art stands in contradiction to Science. It is in part due to the wish to forget the fact that there are large holes in our existing mental health knowledge and that we are often still groping in the dark in our understanding, ability to predict and ability to intervene. Such an admission may lead to the conclusion that this scientific endeavour has not been as successful as the professions may wish to claim. Moreover, it may erode the level of professional confidence and certainty, as well as its public standing.

I would like to argue that when we come to look at the professional activity in mental health — in all disciplines — the dichotomy between Science and Art is false. This is primarily due to the need to apply generalized knowledge to a particular person and a particular situation, where the relationship between the person-in-the-situation and the professional is an additional important component (England, 1986). We are working with people experiencing suffering, confusion and conflict. To assume that this could ever be a simple case of applying scientific knowledge without the need to relate to the person and to attempt to understand and acknowledge underlying factors is an unuseful travesty of reality.

Why enter mental health work?

Putting right a wrong

What attracts us to mental health work? From my personal experience and from the many students and workers I meet regularly, I would dare to suggest that it is a way of putting right a bad experience concerning mental distress, either of ourselves, our close relatives, or friends. It is a form of reparation that has led to the development of a genuine interest in understanding what mental illness is about and in helping people who suffer from it, knowing well that 'there, but for the Grace of God, go I'. At the same time, it is also a form of distancing oneself from being too close to subjective suffering, by having layers of objective and intersubjective knowledge, by relying on procedures of relating to the sufferer and the suffering developed and rehearsed during years of training and work, and by the dulling effect of repeatedly meeting people and situations of intense suffering.

Mental suffering is more difficult to quantify and to understand at both commonsensical and professional levels that is physical illness. Though a common human experience, it is one where the subjective perspective colours the experience to a great degree. Accepting that what is true for most of us is not subjectively true for another person is a very difficult proposition to undertake, yet it is at the foundation of modern understanding of mental distress, even though there may be a disagreement as to the reasons that have led to this state of affairs. The range of interpretation and meaning given to seemingly meaningless experiences and objectively self-defeating behaviour is considerably wide, and one of the tasks of the professional worker is to provide such behaviour with an intelligible meaning.

Risk-taking

The **risk-taking** elements in mental health are always present. They influence our interpretation, categorization, mode of relating to the client, voluntary and involuntary intervention concerning the identified client, relatives and friends. While the issues of life and death are only occasionally at stake (preventing suicide or homicide), often decisions by professionals have a crucial effect on the quality of life of the person for years to come. These decisions are taken with a lower level of certainty than is often the case in relation to physical illness. While this implies the possibility of a creative use of existing knowledge, it may also mean opting for the safest option, even if the latter implies a further reduction in the person's quality of life or his/her future potential for living. Moreover, across the range of interventions the worker herself remains a central instrument of intervention. In part, the attraction in mental health work is that of dealing with the partially unknown, of risking to an extent one's **own** sanity and not only that of one's client, of moving in and out of psychologically threatening territories. It would be difficult to deny that the plight of certain clients, rather than that of equally deserving others, touches us more. Likewise, certain clients antagonize us by behaviour that we are able to tolerate better in others. The possibilities of responding to the client through our personal needs (termed **counter-transference** in psychoanalysis) (Salzberger-Wittenberg, 1978) and obscuring the client's needs therefore require consistent checking in mental health work.

How much of Menzies-Lyth's findings, stated in Table 3.1, is relevant to mental health workers? While the reader is likely to have her own answer to this question, I would like to argue that more of these reactions would typify working in hospitals rather than in community mental health services. Put in another way, I am suggesting that work **setting**, and **support structures** for workers, and not only the subject matter of the work enterprise, have a considerable influence on how we respond as workers.

Job satisfaction

A study on work satisfaction and indicators of burn-out of hospital nurses compared with community psychiatric nurses highlighted that the latter are more satisfied, even though they have higher stress scores (Carson and Bartlett, 1990). Moreover, they were able to retain the interest in the individual client more than hospital nurses. This illustrates that, far from debilitating, taking on personal responsibility and having a multi-task job to perform in a less bureaucratic work environment can be more satisfying professionally and personally.

In another recent and relevant study, Allen *et al.* (1990) have studied two groups of workers in the field of learning difficulties, one hospital-based, the other based in sheltered housing schemes. They were interested in the reactions to being part of a system in transition, as hospitals for people with learning difficulties are closing too. Like Carson and Bartlett, their study was also focused on job satisfaction and stress of the two groups. The findings highlight yet again the higher levels of both satisfaction and stress for workers in the community. In particular, it is illustrated that the latter group of workers is more highly motivated personally and professionally, and is experiencing role ambiguity.

Within the vast range of mental health work individual workers may be more satisfied with one group of clients rather than with another. Evidence from the USA, and from recent British evaluation of demonstration projects in the community, highlights that many mental health workers prefer not to work with continuing care clients and, if left to themselves, opt to work with people with milder levels of distress and better levels of psychosocial functioning (Bachrach, 1983; Patmore, 1987). This is because workers judge the work with the latter group to lead to more positive outcomes. Yet workers in innovative projects with the first group of clients are not less enthusiastic about their work. They have come to expect positive results with a new way of working and to find satisfaction in meeting a challenge, provided they get adequate support (Test and Stein, 1978; Burti and Mosher, 1989). Thus the issue becomes one of balancing expectations for effort with those of satisfaction at outcomes.

Interdisciplinary work in mental health

Rationally, interdisciplinary work is both necessary and attractive to workers. The necessity lies in recognizing that each professional discipline has a contribution to make in leading to positive outcomes for clients, and that pulling together will provide a faster and more comprehensive professional input. The attraction relates to enriching one's understanding and repertoire of interventions by the interdisciplinary exchange, as well as providing mutual support. Both of these elements are central to sustaining mental health workers in the struggle to return people not only to sanity but to ordinary living.

Yet interdisciplinary work is often presented by workers as a major source of conflict and strife, of consistent discontent, as if the gap between the real and the ideal is too big to be bridged.

Much has been said and written about interdisciplinary work, which is not going to be re-stated in this text. The interested reader can look up these sources, beginning with Austin and Hershey (1982), Ovretviet (1986), or Cooper (1990).

It is tempting to suggest that interdisciplinary work has become the convenient peg on which to hang the discomfort of working in mental health, namely to view it as yet another defence mechanism. While there may be some truth in this, as it is safer to blame other professionals than either oneself or one's clients, it might be equally useful to consider other reasons for this sense of being let down by the promise of interdisciplinary work. Perhaps too much has been promised under this heading; perhaps the disciplinary and personal competition is preventing interdisciplinary work from providing a good enough payoff. Alternatively, there are incompatible models at the root of several of the disciplines involved and/or myths about each other that prevent us from being able to work cooperatively, such as the incompatibility of the view of mental illness as an organic disease as opposed to perceiving it as the outcome of failing to resolve basic interpersonal relations and one's sense of personal identity.

Acknowledging what is shared across disciplines, as well as what is not, agreeing on methods of resolving specific conflicts that respect different contributions, can help to reduce tension to a manageable level for many workers. Yet it needs to be recognized that for some workers and for some issues this will be insufficient, and that teams should have the right to choose new members who share the same philosophy. This is especially true in the case of an innovative service, struggling against the understanding of a majority.

To find out more about one aspect of this issue, try out the following exercise, only slightly modified from the original created by Ingrid Barker (1989):

Table 3.2.   Balancing the power

Aim to enable team workers to understand the nature of their own power base, that of other professions, and how it may be used to enhance the power of service users. Also to enable users to understand the extent and limitations of workers' power.

Practicalities
- Allow one-and-a-half hours for this exercise
- A group leader/facilitator is needed
- The group must include a number of service users

Resources
- Flip chart and pens

Table 3.2. *(contd)*

Method
- Divide the group into small groups of two or three people, ensuring that each group has workers from different disciplines and at least one service user
- Ask each member in the group to rate themselves on a scale from 1 to 10 on the power they have over the other participants as workers.
- The group then needs to list those things that are either empowering or disempowering to workers, both in relation to the service they work in and the personal sphere
- Chart the feedback from each small group onto a collective flip chart-sized sheet
- Repeat the small group exercise of power rating, but from the perspective of other disciplines and that of service users in the group
- Chart the feedback onto a collective flip chart
- Discuss the issues raised, particularly linking those areas where users' power can be enhanced by workers' abilities to help (e.g. when users wish to run their own drop-in centre, workers may be able to help by seeking funding). It is also important to recognize that some myths may have been challenged during the exercise (e.g. the power of different disciplines, that workers are all-powerful while users are completely powerless)

Adapted from Barker (1990).

This exercise reminds us that issues of power are not limited to the interdisciplinary dimension — users' relative power or lack of it and the powers of the organization in which we are working are additional components of the equation of power. The issue of users' involvement in hospital closure is discussed in the next section.

HOSPITAL CLOSURE: ISSUES FOR PROFESSIONAL WORKERS
IN THE HOSPITAL

Issues around the decision to close a hospital

The decision to close hospitals in principle, and the decision to close a particular hospital, is invariably experienced as a shock to the workers. This is partly because it implies a considerable departure from the known to the unknown, and partly because it signifies failure to provide a good enough mental health facility. Both factors present the staff with considerable ambivalence, and for some with straightforward conflict, crisis and hostility. The first factor is more general to any fundamental organizational change, ranging from commercial business enterprises to introducing changes in agriculture, which affect the lives of millions of people. Handling it well includes components such as involving those who are going to be most affected by the change as much as possible in both the preparatory thinking about it and in carrying it out.

'Breaking the news' in a disarming yet honest way is another important variable, which should be well known to any mental health worker who has been engaged in telling clients directly, and their relatives, about the significance of the specific difficulties and mental distress/illness that they may suffer from. Yet in a London hospital much studied in relation to closure processes, staff first learned about its proposed closure from local and national newspapers. When finally formally told by the management, the announcement lacked details of staff deployment prospects. Such a strategy is sure to backfire in getting staff support for the closure.

Compare this with the approach of the health authority in Exeter, which first negotiated a no-redundancy agreement with the local trade unions prior to announcing the intended closure of its psychiatric hospitals (King, 1991). Or compare this with the likely effect on staff support of the resignation of all senior professional staff from the psychiatric hospital in Gorizia, northern Italy, in 1967, in protest against being let down by the province's administration over promised resources for hospital closure, made public first to all staff and hospital residents, and then to the administration and the general public (Tranchina and Basaglia, 1979).

Compare further with experiences in Arezzo, Trieste and Turin in which patients and staff were meeting daily for more than a year to discuss how they would like to change the hospital and to monitor the agreed changes, *prior* to any discussion of hospital closure (De Nicola, 1991; Basaglia, 1968). This had a dual effect of not only securing a greater readiness by the staff towards approaching fundamental change in a positive light, but also of **demonstrating** to them that they have a valid contribution to make that is taken on board and implemented. In such a context, the decision to close the hospital came as a natural progression from the changes that were already underway and in which staff were active and valued participants. Therefore there was no need for the staff to be defensive or to feel that their whole way of working and their professional identity were discarded, even though central elements of it were criticized. This is not to imply that there were no conflicts, no disagreements, or bitter exchanges of words (and even flour bombs between staff and staff, to the amazement and amusement of the patients ...!) in these Italian experiences. Nevertheless, there was an atmosphere in which these could be expressed, worked through, and resolved in one way or another.

These examples illustrate that **there is a range of ways** in which breaking the news to the staff (and to others) and planning a participatory ensuing process of work can lead to positive responses to the challenge of closure.

The implied criticism in the decision to close a hospital

A decision to close a hospital signifies agreement with the assumption that hospitals are not the preferred mode of working with people suffering from mental illness. While arguments for and against the closure of psychiatric hospitals have been presented in the Introduction of this book, in this section it is intended to look at the implications for professional workers of the decision to close a hospital.

Workers who have been persuaded by the arguments for closure will find it easier to accept such a decision than workers who have not been persuaded. However, both groups will have to come to terms with the inherent critique of the hospital as the primary intervention site to which they have all contributed. No one likes to be given the impression that they have participated in a devalued enterprise, or to feel blamed and guilty for their professional contribution — especially if individual workers feel that they have given the job their best, or were prevented from doing so by factors beyond their control.

A whole range of **defensive arguments** come to the fore, some more realistic and weighty than others, when a hospital closure is announced. The undeniable lack of sufficient services in the community and the risk of neglect to long-term residents of the psychiatric hospitals, should they be made to leave, have been cited in defence of maintaining hospitals. Such statements are made while omitting to mention that hospitals consume two-thirds of the budget for psychiatric services in most Western countries, yet treat less than a quarter of the population that suffers from mental health difficulties. Such statements omit to mention also that the majority of those who use the hospital live for most of the time outside it — 60% of all British admissions to psychiatric hospitals last for no more than one month; another 20% for up to three months (HPSSS, 1991).

It has been argued that the hospital has become home for this group of people that has been excluded from ordinary living for so long. This is claimed without pausing to ask what has led to their exclusion and whether their hospitalization has secured not only the exclusion but the lack of skills to re-enter ordinary living, and how they respond when given a real and supported opportunity to move out (see Chapter Four). This issue has been taken on board positively, in solutions such as converting wards to ordinary, yet supported, housing schemes on the premises of a closed hospital (Del Giudice, 1991; Glynn, 1991).

Defensive tactics include blaming other professional groups than one's own — the hospital administration, the Health Authority, the Government, the community. A different set of tactics has been both the intentional and largely unintentional sabotage of the work aimed directly at closing the hospital, making the lives of special teams responsible for closure as difficult as possible, and refusing to accept that the hospital will close. Others have responded by securing transfers to other hospitals or an early transfer to a community service, while others moved to the commercial sector as self-employed entrepreneurs.

Variations in the responses of professional groups

The wholesale closure of psychiatric hospitals in the USA and in Italy clearly adhered to the view that non-hospital treatment is to be preferred to hospital treatment in terms of rehabilitation prospects, and economic and personal costs. To reach this conclusion, it was necessary to go through the phase of denouncing the ills of hospital-based intervention, invariably touching upon issues such as professional contribution, and attributing more responsibility, and blame, to some professions rather than to others. Psychiatrists and nurses were the two professions singled out for this, the first as the leaders and the second as the largest group of professional workers. Psychiatrists in the USA and in Britain have responded by defending the hospitals and defending their own practice, by bidding to gain more power in the services (in Britain), or by leaving the new public services altogether (in the USA), rather than by re-examining or changing their ways of working and thinking.

Facing work in the community as a challenge

Nurses in both countries have responded by creating a new speciality, namely that of community psychiatric nursing (CPN), which sees itself as providing a very different contribution to clients and to multidisciplinary teams than hospital nurses (Brooker, 1990; White, 1990). In fact, in Britain many of the CPNs have never worked in the hospital. I would argue that this solution to the burden of blame, guilt and the doubts related to professional identity has several clear advantages, but also some more covert disadvantages. The advantages include the enthusiasm and sense of mission that comes with a new field of activities and identity, the exhilaration of learning new skills which seem to offer a better service, of feeling appreciated by the clients and by workers from other disciplines.

The disadvantage is that this solution of distancing a group from the professional collective and re-creating a new professional identity for the subgroup is costly. The price is paid, in particular, by the many hospital nurses who are left to carry the brunt of the blame and guilt without the prospect of redemption.

Facing hospital closure as a challenge

An alternative solution took place in several places in Italy, where all of the nurses working in hospitals participated firstly in the process of transforming the hospital into a better living setting and, secondly, moved to work in the community. Through this two-stage process they had the opportunity to work out for themselves what were the negative and the positive areas of their approach and ways of working, what were the desirable alternatives, and how to reach the new balance themselves. By being able to be active in this process they demonstrated to others and to themselves the capacity to effect change and the ability to unlearn and relearn. For that they have earned the respect of their colleagues, their clients and their families, as well as self-respect (Battaglia, 1987; De Nicola, 1991).

Likewise, a sizable minority of Italian psychiatrists took the criticisms seriously, in fact generating the critique and the local and national Italian reform that has followed on from their position. While the main points of their critique have been mentioned in the Introduction to this book, the focus in this section is on how they have handled it in their everyday work, as well as in planning the new mental health system.

The psychiatrists, who were unhappy with the mental health system that they inherited, joined ranks with like-minded nurses and social workers to rethink what they would like to see instead and how it could be implemented, rather than retaining their dominant but isolated position. Considerable self-criticism was expressed, which was not paralleled by the outside world. Perhaps because there was no pressure from the outside, the self-criticism may have developed with less recourse to defensive tactics. Their thinking was influenced by the general social context, certain schools of French and Italian philosophy, sociology, and Anglo Saxon social psychiatry, but above all by their own practice wisdom and that of the patients. This self-criticism led to the rejection of the controlling role of professional practice as much as possible and the **re-discovery** of the interpersonal **affinity** with the clients as human beings, including the wish to restore subjectivity and self-respect to the patients. It also led to rejecting many of the techniques of intervention which were seen as unsuitable in the light of critique (such as electroconvulsive shock treatment), yet retaining some others, notably medication. The use of medication highlights some of the ambiguities remaining in a reformed psychiatric system, as the Italian professionals are aware of the side-effects of medication and of the power over the client that its use gives to the professional. Nevertheless, the essence of the thrust for a reformed system was on constructing new organizational structures in which to practise what has been perceived to be an improved mental health system.

The focus on **organizational change,** which came in Italy from within the professions, was related to the recognition of the campaigning role that professionals have to undertake if they wish to implement structural change. Thus networking, acting as a pressure group, carrying out political work yet without becoming aligned to any one political party, became accepted as a necessity in which all professionals needed to engage.

Psichiatria Democratica. In 1976, more than ten years after the first experiment with changing the system, the workers created an umbrella movement, called Psichiatria Democratica, a movement of professionals around the single issue of the reform (Ramon, 1983; Crepet, 1983; Tranchina and Basaglia, 1979). With this phase, the professional identity of the worker — a nurse, a social worker, or a psychiatrist — has completed a 'sea-change', from being a technician (a term used derogatively by Italian colleagues) serving the controlling forces within society to that of the liberator interested in forming new, closer and more supportive relations with the client on the one hand, and a political change agent in relation to the general public on the other. This image of self (and others) perhaps overlooks the controlling aspects of work in the community, but is quite accurate in relation to the work in the hospital during the closure process.

By 1991, Psichiatria Democratica did not seem to exist as a national professional movement any more, although some local branches continued to function. Was this outcome due to the end of its historical mission, namely the focus on hospital closure? Has it been replaced by obtaining and retaining political power (e.g. through the election of MPs with similar views)? Alternatively, it highlights perhaps the weakness of basing a professional movement on one issue without securing a continuous basis for its existence as a school of thought (e.g. no long-term training structure or research was organized by this movement). Still further its demise may signify that the membership had become tired and less enthusiastic, and/or that campaigning for community services, which did not have a concrete symbol such as the hospital, mobilized people less.

The British and Australian message differs somewhat in that not all psychiatric hospitals are to be closed. This may be taken to imply that the reason for clousure is one of economic consideration only. Indeed, many professionals in these countries have taken this to mean that it does not imply any criticism about their ways of working, and all that is required from them is a physical relocation. While seemingly less critical of hospital treatment, such a direction helps to obscure the issue of why it is necessary to close psychiatric hospitals and prevents professionals from re-examining their ways of working.

Cultural variations seem to matter in opting for specific solutions to the issue of the inherent criticism of workers. Yet, in each culture, there are solutions that embrace the challenging aspects of the closure, in contrast to those that embrace the more defensive aspects. Groups of workers, as well as individuals, have therefore a measure of choice as to which type of solution they wish to opt for.

Working out the principal objectives of hospital closure and the best ways of their attainment

On the surface, the aim of hospital closure is deceptively simple, namely not to have hospitals as the primary site of mental health intervention. However, this encapsulates also the following:

1. Preparing the residents for life outside the hospital;

2. Preparing the staff for work outside the hospital, as well as to support residents in their preparation;
3. Preparing local communities and local services for the move;
4. When necessary, preparing new workers for supporting residents and hospital staff.

While the first objective is the prime concern, all three others are essential ingredients in the attempt to attain it, as each objective/facet is interdependent on the others.

For example, consider the effect on the hospital workforce of introducing a transitional team from the outside. This signifies the message that the hospital staff cannot prepare residents for their lives outside and cannot be redeployed in the new services. It immediately puts the hospital staff on the defensive, leading to hostility, apathy, sabotage, and self-defeatist behaviour. Instead, the hospital management can do one of the following: (a) encourage all workers to revamp rehabilitation procedures and engage in changing the hospital to fit with the new procedures; or (b) provide extra training for a core, interdisciplinary, group of workers to start a pilot project within the hospital, using it as a demonstration project for the rest of the staff who will also get the extra training in their turn. I would argue that either of these strategies would lead to treating the closure as a challenge, rather than as a threat, mobilizing the workforce to work **for** closure, rather than against it. Indeed, the good examples of the Italian psychiatric reform demonstrate such an approach.

Working towards the move of most residents to live outside the hospital and working on preparing the local community require additional sets of skills to those usually required for work in the most liberal psychiatric hospital, or in preparing individually one resident at a time for a similar move. Considerable organizational skills, group and community work skills are then in demand. Yet these are the very skills that are either left out of the training curriculum of most helping professions or taught at no more than beginners' level.

Froland's list (Table 3.3) is much longer; most of it focuses on work in the community. However, there is nothing to prevent workers in hospital from

Table 3.3. What community work can offer to mental health work

Problem focus	Mental health clients
Individual rights	
Access to services	Develop pool of volunteers
Acceptability and	to help obtain services for
appropriateness	returning hospital patients
Stigmatizing problems	Organize consumers advocacy,
	advice or self-help groups

Table 3.3.   *(contd)*

Problem focus	Mental health clients
Needs for material assistance	
Food	Establish citizen/consumer partnership
Housing	to organize employment and housing
Jobs	opportunities for this group
Needs for social and emotional support	
Limitations in social skills	Develop networks among ex-patients to initiate and plan social and recreational activities

Adapted from Froland (1981).

applying the principle and the methods to work in the hospital. Befriending schemes between volunteers from the community and people in hospital are one such application; a group of young black people in hospital planning outings together is another application that I have come across. More ambitious but achievable initiatives are residents' newspapers (Basaglia, 1968) and the Dutch and British patients' councils described in the next section or the users' forum described by Wainwright in Chapter One of this book.

Appreciation and basic understanding of non-clinical areas of work also becomes indispensable, such as housing, income support, working with volunteers, informal and formal networks in the community, even if focused work in these areas will be carried out by specialists. Furthermore, creating the necessary conditions for the innovation that is required for the many small and large changes in service organization and service delivery. The skills with which to establish these conditions too are not taught as part of professional training.

The necessary conditions for innovation:

1. Shared dissatisfaction with the status quo;
2. Shared vision of the future and aims for change;
3. Knowledge about 'first practical steps';
4. Economic and psychological costs for people must not be greater than the three points above;
5. Organization operates in goal-directed mode;
6. Decision-making is based on who is close to the issue, rather than position in role or hierarchy;
7. Reward systems are related to work to be done;
8. Communication is relatively open;
9. Collaboration is rewarded;
10. The organization is seen as an open system;

11. Individuality and individuals are valued; and
12. 'Action-research' mode of management, incorporating feedback systems for monitoring.

These were adapted from an NHS training authority (NHSTA) White Hart internal document.

Opportunities for collective users' participation in hospital closure

While Chapter Four will discuss the opportunities, or lack of them, for involving individual clients in hospital closure, I would like to suggest that there is a valid and useful place for collective involvement of users in this process. The validity is based on the objectives of mental health work, especially those of hospital closure, which are about supporting people in overcoming the impact of mental illness and in regaining abilities and the respect required for ordinary living. The ability to contribute to a collective effort is worthwhile encouraging within such a perspective. The usefulness relates to the observation that people who feel involved in a process develop a greater commitment to its success, as has been stressed in relation to the staff group.

In turn, the commitment of the residents supports also the staff, as the latter depend for job satisfaction in part on the achievements of the first group. An interesting example is provided by patients, councils that exist in Holland and in some British towns — in 40 out of the 43 Dutch hospitals and in Bristol, London, Nottingham and Newcastle (NGA, 1989). In these situations, ex-patients act as the initial organizers of ward meetings in which patients are encouraged to express their views and discuss, without staff presence, alternatives to services that they find unsatisfactory. These meetings gradually become forums run by the ward residents, who thus also gain access to information and communication with the hospital management. Although not used so far in conjunction with hospital closure, such a council can become a vehicle to offer feedback to the management concerning the closure process, as well as to encourage the partnership of the hospital residents in the process. The users' forum described by Wainwright in Chapter One illustrates how effective such a collective involvement can be in achieving specific aims such as bolstering the self-image and representation skills of long-term residents in psychiatric hospitals.

In Arezzo, during the re-organization of the hospital as part of the closure process, long-term patients have learned to contribute to the staff-residents meetings, and eventually chaired these meetings, which became a major body of internal decision-making.

Constructing alternatives to hospital-focused intervention

The closure of hospitals accentuates the need to establish alternative services. Given the multiplicity of the tasks and the variety of participants, the thinking, planning and construction of these alternatives should be a shared process. The case study to follow in this chapter, and all of the other chapters in this book provide plenty of evidence to suggest that this has not been the case in Britain.

In Italy, the users and the general public had more of a say in specific instances (Pirella, 1982) but the planning has remained largely in the professional and administrative domains. American mandatory advisory boards and experimentation with users and relatives representation on planning groups in a few British neighbourhoods (e.g. North Derbyshire, Hackney, Lambeth) illustrate some of the largely untapped possibilities for a more participatory process of planning.

However, even in a more fully participative process, professionals will continue to have a leading role in constructing alternative services, as they are likely either to work directly in these services or provide guidance to other care staff. Hence the centrality of professionals in planning future services is to remain.

While each professional worker may have his/her own ideas concerning alternative services and use these to influence the development of local services, we usually look to our professional associations and the Ministry of Health to provide us with a more comprehensive perspective. It is no secret that the Ministry too asks for the views of professional associations, as one component among several that the Civil Service and the political leadership will take into account in their deliberations.

Surprisingly little has been offered by the different professional associations in the countries where psychiatric hospitals have closed on a large scale. No professional association of the five major disciplines (nursing, occupational therapy, clinical psychology, psychiatry and social work) in Australia, Britain, Italy and the USA has addressed hospital closure as an issue of professional concern and debate in a publication focused on hospital closure. Only one British nursing trade union, the Confederation of Health Service Employees (COHSE) has twice produced publications that pay systematic attention to hospital closure and not only to community services (COHSE, 1983, 1991). However, while both publications focus on crucial issues such as financial resources, they fail to take into account the full implications of closure for the role of the nurse. The Psichiatria Democratica movement already mentioned was the response of the Italian professionals, but similar (but considerably smaller in scale and influence) movements in Germany and Brazil, inspired by the Italians, have remained the exceptions (Harlin, 1987; Vasconcelos, 1991).

Professional associations too are focusing exclusively on arrangements for clients, forgetting their brief not only to defend professional interests but also to provide leadership in a time of questioning professional knowledge, skills, and roles. The fact that they can so easily put aside this task would imply that there is not much pressure from among their rank-and-file members to provide leadership in relation to the closure, either because members do not have much faith in their associations or because they too prefer not to confront the issues raised by the closure. The emphasis on services in the community, the denial of the link between hospital closure and these services, the lack of attention to the **processes** involved in closure for the professional and for the hospital as a live organism, seem to be shared by workers, their associations and the administrators. Inevitably, this omission leads to further isolation of hospital workers, who are expected somehow to move on their own from the hospital and its mentality to services in the community and their mentality. However, such a strategy is not only self-defeating and costly for the professional identity of those working in hospitals. It also prevents a much needed re-examination of what are the objectives of mental health services, where have services and professionals gone wrong in the past, and how this can be put right in the new services.

The North American experience

An example in point is the North American experience of wholesale hospital closures, which is often mentioned in Europe as a total failure. Indicators of failure include the number of homeless people who suffer from mental illness, prisoners with mental illness, and the reluctance of mental health workers to work with the continued care client (Lamb, 1990; Bachrach, 1983). Neither the indicators nor the commentators themselves relate to the process of hospital closure, or the quality of life in the new mini-hospital facilities that were established instead. Again, the total denial of this component would seem to reflect the discomfort that is likely to be faced without the denial.

It is worth our while to know a little about these facilities, as in Europe we need to ask ourselves whether we would like to have them too, and our American colleagues need to ask themselves whether this is a system worthwhile retaining, or whether we all need urgently to look for other alternatives. The 'closed facilities' as they are known contain up to 100 people, mostly between the ages of 25–40, for up to one year. They are owned by large commercial corporations, which also own many nursing homes, and indeed they look like nursing homes. Most of the care staff are unqualified, with one year post high-school training, leading to the title 'psychiatric technician'. A mixture of medication and rehabilitative activities appear on the formal programme, but observations indicate that the reliance on medication is considerable and that either many of the scheduled activities do not take place or the residents do not join in. The reward for good behaviour and participation in activities is to be accompanied out of the facility for a specified time. Indeed, it would be difficult to justify hospital closure if such facilities would be the only alternative.

Considerably fewer in number are North American facilities, such as Cedar House in Boulder, where people in a psychotic episode can take refuge, be offered medication and counselling, as well as participation in the everyday activities of the home. The home is in fact a house in a middle-class area, which is pleasantly furnished and not locked (Warner, 1991).

Alternative asylum facilities

Even less known to the Anglo-Saxon professionals are existing alternative asylum facilities in a place like Trieste, where all mental health centres have beds and in which they take care of people in an acute mental breakdown as well as at all other stages, with an impressive track record of a very low number of suicides, homicides, compulsory admissions to this open facility and also length of either compulsory or voluntary admissions (Sain *et al.*, 1990). This re-opens the debate as to what were the objectives of hospital treatment, as well as where have those been met or not, and the reasons for the inability to satisfactorily meet objectives in the hospital.

Often it is assumed that hospitals were there to offer **asylum,** a refuge or a haven from the pressures generated by ordinary living. We need to ask ourselves whether this has been offered positively or negatively, as prison too is an asylum but not the type of refuge that we would describe as a haven. When listening to users' descriptions of their experience, it is the constraining aspects that come through (see Chapter Four). These included the regimentation, the lack of choice, of privacy, of home-like atmosphere, the noise and lack of tranquillity (Ramon, 1990), which are also documented by Wainwright in Chapter One. Having ascertained that often hospitals have failed to offer asylum, we need to consider the construction of asylum facilities in the community to ensure that they will indeed offer an improved refuge opportunity, one in which tranquillity and easing of pressures exist side by side with choice and the gradual re-assuming of ordinary life responsibilities.

Preparing residents to re-enter ordinary life

The second main caring task of hospitals has been to prepare residents to **re-enter ordinary life**. The accounts provided in Chapter Four, the passivity that has typified life in psychiatric hospital would indicate that this objective too has not been satisfactorily achieved. However, it could be argued that this could never have been a goal to be achieved by the hospital on its own, but in conjunction with services outside it. The passivity that was fostered in hospitals has been often justified as either the result of the illness and the effect of the medication, or as a means to ensure social control over a deviant group.

There is agreement among both professionals and users that, during the most acute phase of a mental breakdown, people find it difficult, if not impossible, to handle everyday responsibilities. There is no such agreed agenda for the post-acute phase, or for the level and duration of the use of medication. In fact, the issue of the continuous use of medication is one of the major 'bones of contention' between users' organizations and the medical profession, and between social workers and doctors. There is evidence to suggest that when asylum is offered in the community or in an environment that encourages shared activity (e.g. therapeutic community) a considerably lower level of passivity is observed and a quicker return to a more ordinary lifestyle is made possible (Burti and Mosher, 1989).

The social-control function

The **controlling function** of mental health services, and of the mental health professionals who lead the services, is usually ignored by them and/or justified as a therapeutic necessity. The closure of psychiatric hospitals has been campaigned under the banner of care, and as means of ensuring the end of the controlling function. I would like to suggest that while most services in the community exercise a lower level of coercive social control they continue to function as social control agents. Therefore this function should be acknowledged and examined as an element of the role of mental health professionals. The controlling part is performed through every professional task, from that of giving meaning to mental distress, through the assessment of the level of distress, decisions about degree of risk, type of intervention, predictions about the future ('prognosis') and about people's potential. The controlling feature is inevitable (given the social mandate of professionals) and is socially desirable in terms of defending acceptable norms of rationality and propriety, danger to oneself and to others.

Related to hospital closure, it is the task of the planners to take into account the social-control function and to devise new structures that 'take it on board', without the creation of mini prisons in the community. There is sufficient evidence to ascertain that 'soft' (i.e. less coercive) measures of control, such as counselling and living in staffed, sheltered accommodation, are more effective as deterrents of socially undesirable behaviour than coercive measures such as compulsory admission (Castel *et al.*, 1982; Miller and Rose, 1986). However, professionals used to coercive measures would need to go through considerable unlearning and relearning processes to be able to use effectively the less coercive measures. A gradual process of hospital closure, in which professionals are encouraged to use soft measures of control in what feels like a 'safe' environment to them and to the users, is the ideal setting for such a transformation, as the good example of the Italian reform has demonstrated.

Nevertheless, soft measures can be as abused as coercive measures are at times. Quality control mechanisms, if used tactfully, can help, as can adequate peer support and supervision, to reduce the risk. The more participatory the management style, the more say users have in the way a facility is run, the more likely it is that only soft measures would be used and the less likely that they will be over-used. However, as users who manage services have discovered to their chagrin, they too need to resort to some measures of social control, such as a constitution concerning membership that permits the expulsion of members in extreme circumstances.

MAKING SENSE OF THE EXPERIENCE OF CLOSURE: A CASE STUDY OF SOCIAL WORK TEAMS

Why focus on social work?

British social workers have embraced community mental health ideas more readily than other professions in the past (Ramon, 1985a). Yet any reader of social work popular journals, or anyone bothering to talk to social workers, cannot but be aware of the current apprehension among them of the inappropriate application of these ideas (due to the combination of inadequate resources, the paucity of supportive services in an indifferent community, and the dominance of the clinical-somatic approaches to mental illness in the psychiatric services). Being much more used to working in the community than most other professional groups, social workers have been, and hopefully will continue to be, a crucial group in the provision of community services for people with mental illness. In a world less controlled by the artificial divide of 'health' and 'social' care needs and budgets, social workers would have been the ideal spearheading group of the change entailed in introducing community mental health. With the new British legislation, the NHS and Community Care Bill (1990), which came into effect in relation to mental health in April 1991 and April 1993, their role is likely to be both re-examined and redefined in some central aspects. Therefore it is important and timely to study how social workers face the closure of the hospital in which they are working.

In one of the very few studies of professionals facing a major reorganization, Carol Satyamurti (1982) looked at the reactions of social workers to the introduction of generic teams in the early 1970s in a British town, and has illustrated the predominantly defensive nature of their response. The studies by Menzies-Lyth (1988), Carson and Bartlett (1990), and Allen *et al* (1990), already described earlier in this chapter, focused either on the defences employed by clinical staff or on job satisfaction and stresses experienced by individual workers.

While these are important dimensions in closure work, to approach the latter study primarily as another instance of individualized work stress would be to apply a reductionist perspective of this group process and its significance for the workforce. Within this study, the closure was approached as a process that entails potential challenge, threat, crisis and innovation for the professionals involved in it. More specifically, it was hypothesized that when this process is meaningful, it should result in a re-examination of professional knowledge, skills, and identity, eventually leading to a modification of content and methods of work. In the light of this approach, and in the absence of knowledge gained from relevant studies, the following research questions were formulated:

1. How is closure work defined?
2. How and why are decisions on closure work reached?
3. What are the views of the social workers concerning the closure, their place within the mental health system, their views of the ideal mental health system?
4. What are the views of key others of social work involvement in mental health, and in particular concerning the role of social workers in the closure process?
5. Have the closure process and the closure work influenced professional knowledge, skills, and identity?

To summarize, this study focused on the relationships among organization change, management styles, and professional roles in the context of closure work for social workers.

Methodology

In the absence of closely related research, or even a relevant information base, the methodology had to be invented from scratch to enable the author to attempt to answer the questions mentioned. Thus the research tools had to capture the descriptive, attitudinal and analytic information. A research strategy that is qualitative in essence, and which enables subjective views to emerge side by side with a team perspective, had to be developed. Given these requirements, methodological triangulation became a necessity (Smith and Cantly, 1985).

Three social-work teams working in the same psychiatric hospital but each for a different local authority were studied. In addition, seven key people external to the teams were interviewed: three were consultant psychiatrists responsible for the Health District's wards corresponding to the three local authorities, the hospital General Unit Manager, and the three Social Service Assistant Directors who were managerially responsible for the teams. One interdisciplinary team was also observed, as it evolved in response to the closure work process.

Semi-structured interviews with individual team members and several key people from other disciplines, the hospital management and the management of each Social Services department formed one tool, aimed at gaining information and attitudinal views. Individual team members were interviewed twice, to get a measure of the change in their views and attitudes. Repeated interviews meant that key items had to be phrased differently or approached in stylistically different ways, such as open-ended questions in the first interview and a vignette on the same issue in the second interview.

Observation of team meetings and writing down their content took place weekly for 18 months, providing rich information on the content and process of decision-making in relation to closure. The information related to the policy aspects and the planning process at the Health and Social Services management levels, described in Chapter Two (and in greater details in Tomlinson, 1991), was very useful as background knowledge. The author participated in several interdisciplinary management planning meetings for her to become better acquainted with the planning process and its content.

The empirical study took place between March 1987 and September 1988, at the middle phase of the closure process. Only the main findings of the research will be outlined and only one major issue, that of a culture of innovation, will be looked at in the light of the findings.

The context

The hospital in which the study took place was due for closure in 1993; it had 800 patients in 1987, while it housed, in its 'heyday', 2000 people. In July 1990, it was announced that it would close two years earlier, namely in 1991, a decision further modified to September 1992. It was a teaching hospital that was well known for its medical treatment, rather than for a psychosocial emphasis, although it had a well-developed industrial workshop. The closure was decided on financial grounds by the Regional Health Authority; many of the psychiatrists and nurses objected to it and have attempted to reverse the decision in a variety of ways.

The full complement of each of the three social-work teams consisted of six workers and a team leader; one team had also a principal social worker, who was responsible not only for this group of workers. Decision-making processes within the teams were fairly democratic, whereas the managing style from headquarters in two of the three departments was characterized by decisions handed from above, with little or no discussion. Two of the Social Services departments were going through a considerable financial and managerial crisis during the study period. All three boroughs had been rate-capped, and later charge-capped (namely penalized by the Government for assumed over-spending by a cut in their allocation from Central Government). All three boroughs had a mixture of affluent and poor areas, as well as several ethnic minority groups. Two of the boroughs were noted in the 1970s for well-developed welfare services.

During the study, the membership of one team changed completely; the membership of a second team was reduced to one full-time social worker, and the membership of the third team was short of three workers. In part, it was difficult to retain workers and attract new ones of the right professional calibre to a place due for closure and to a department in crisis; in part, the departments took their time to re-advertise and interview in an insecure financial climate. In addition, there were no formal links or organized meetings among the three teams, in contrast to the existence of such links among psychiatrists and nurses. This is but one example of the lack of formal support systems.

Closure work was defined as work with people who had been in hospital for more than two years. This implies that the major component of the social workers' load, that is work with people in the acute wards, was not perceived as closure work, even though most of it is focused on discharge from hospital. This definition, and the lack of financial support for the rehabilitation of people in acute wards outside the hospital, highlights a rather short-sighted policy that was lacking in preventive objectives and likely to contribute to the creation of a new group of long-term service users. Initial decisions concerning closure plans arose out of a joint planning process of Health and Social Services; all of the additional resources for closure work coming out of the Health Authorities' budgets or joint funding.

Long-stay residents were to be prepared in the hospital, in terms of self care and social skills necessary for the move to sheltered accommodation in small groups outside it, and to attend day centres. Accommodation was to be provided mainly by voluntary organizations, as were some of the day centres. Other day centres were managed by the Social Services departments.

Closure work

This took a different form in each team. One team did not do any, due to a decision taken by the local branch of the trade union NALGO that, unless additional workers were appointed for closure work, no social worker should do it. The two team members who were keen to go ahead with this type of work found themselves censored by the rest of the team, and had to stop any clear involvement in such work. The Social Services department established a rehabilitation centre outside the hospital, as part of its joint planning with the Health Authority, thus largely by-passing the social work team and the decision taken by NALGO. Several multidisciplinary community mental health centres were 'in the pipeline', based on the assumption of employing new social workers, rather than those who were then based in the hospital. The Health District also decided to have a unit with 120 beds on the site of the psychiatric hospital. Plans also existed for group homes and housing associations, and an adult placements scheme was in operation.

The second team allocated two newly appointed social workers to be attached for most of their working week to the multidisciplinary team set up at one area of the Authority to prepare hospital residents for the move into the community, whose salaries were paid by the Health Authority. Although they were inundated with requests to support the residential homes being established by the voluntary sector, the rest of the team did not carry out closure work, because they were understaffed. The multidisciplinary specialist team operated in the area of the District that managed the hospital. Several staffed group homes were 'on stream' or 'in the pipeline'; 60 additional beds were to be added to the local General Hospital, which had already a Day Hospital and a psychiatric ward.

The third team opted for the involvement of each team member in at least one closure project, after experimenting with leaving it to two workers only. Members of this team were involved in initiatives such as running a preparatory group for black young male patients, setting up several new group homes to be run by voluntary organizations, a planning group for a General Hospital unit for people with special needs, beside their participation in multidisciplinary assessment of each long-term resident. An active and innovative senior social worker, whose post was financed by the Health Authority, was responsible at Borough level for closure projects. Several group homes were already functioning, while others were at different stages of the planning process.

The Health District of the third team established a transitional team consisting of nurses and psychologists aimed also at preparing individual residents for the move into the community. Despite good working relationships between the Health and Social Services in this case, it is significant that the authority did not wish to have Local Authority social workers attached to this team. Ironically, the person appointed to lead the team was a qualified social worker, heading a team with a nursing background. Similarly, plans for running a mental health resource centre were based on excluding Local Authority social workers from the core team. A unit for people with special needs was to be established within the nearest General Hospital, together with a psychogeriatric unit. That hospital had already a psychiatric wing, with a day hospital.

The psychiatric hospital had (and still has) a research unit focused on the closure process. Tellingly, social workers have not been involved in this venture, neither as researchers, consultants to research projects, participants, nor as subjects of research. The joint planning process is studied from a social policy perspective, and has not looked at the involvement of 'grass-root' workers in this process.

Team members' views on the closure

All social workers welcomed the closure, based on their wish to see residents de-segregated and offered a more psychosocial intervention. With one exception of a worker who welcomed the benefit of the hospital's grounds for patients' relaxation, no positive comment was made about the hospital. Nearly all commented on their sense of being marginalized in the hospital by other disciplines as the main frustrating element of the work there, while joining a multidisciplinary team was one of the major initial reasons for working in the hospital.

Each worker could suggest several individual staff members from other disciplines whose work they respected, and no worker was against medical intervention. Yet, on the whole, they felt that clients were not treated with the respect they deserved or with the right mixture of intervention methods, citing examples where unilateral decisions were taken by medical staff without consultation with either social worker or patient, and changes in joint work practices implemented without even informing social workers of these changes.

The Consultants' and the General Unit Manager's views were that the contribution of social workers was important, but could be provided perhaps by other workers, such as nurses. While some of them thought that social workers should offer more welfare advice and sort out practical difficulties, one consultant felt strongly that social workers should offer more counselling than they were providing.

Concerning closure work, the two teams whose members were involved in it thought that the direction was, on the whole, positive but were apprehensive about the continuing dominance of the medical view on the one hand, and the delays in implementation by both health and social services on the other. Some members of the third team were less content with the direction of closure plans for their area, which included retaining 120 beds on the site of the psychiatric hospital, already mentioned.

Most workers were aware of the unintentional sabotage of closure work by ward staff who were unhappy with the closure. For example, although half of the hospital was empty, the new core team was not offered proper office space or a space in which to do group work with residents for quite some time. Bets were taken in wards as to how long would 'resident X' manage to remain outside before the 'inevitable' breakdown. It is not too difficult to imagine that this message was conveyed to the resident, increasing the likelihood of a self-fulfilling prophecy materializing.

When asked about the **ideal service** they would like to see, workers suggested a system in which **genuine** multidisciplinary mental health centres would be the backbone, supported by psychiatric wards in general hospitals, group homes and day centres. They were particularly critical of the current day centres, seen to foster passivity and offer irrelevant activities. The terms 'genuine' or 'true' multidisciplinary work (which were not introduced by the researcher) were repeatedly stressed by the participants. By 'genuine', workers meant the acceptance by all of the participants in such teams of the valued contribution provided by each discipline and the ability to work in a way that reflected this acceptance. With the exception of the last point, this view of the future was similar to that expressed by the consultants, and is far from the more radical perspective taken by social workers who, at the time of writing, were initiating the involvement of users in the planning and the running of services, self-help and advocacy initiatives (Barker and Peck, 1987; Milroy and Hennelly, 1989). This is not to say that team members opposed these relatively new directions, but they were not active in pursuing them and did not see them as essential in the future system.

Towards a culture of innovation?

Five years after the formal decision to close the hospital and well into the process of closure with patients leaving it, a culture that actively encouraged and fostered innovative change did not emerge. There were no signs that the closure process had influenced significantly the views and methods of working of two out of the three teams, while it has influenced the work of the third team in part. This comment should not be read to imply that the work done was not good but that, in a major change process such as a hospital closure, reassessment of past work and innovation would be expected, with methods of work to follow suit.

I would like to stress that the relative lack of innovation highlighted in this study stood in contrast to the commitment, intelligence and liveliness of individual team members. It is therefore all the more necessary to consider factors that would militate against innovation.

Marginalization within the hospital

The **marginalization within the hospital** was one of the more obvious factors. When a group of workers feels marginalized and undervalued, it is unlikely to innovate in areas of joint work. This marginalization requires attention as to its reasons, if it is to be reduced in the future, both inside and outside the hospitals. Within the hospital, there were both structural and ideological reasons leading to this alienation; only some of the structural elements will disappear outside the hospital. Yet, even within the closing hospitals there are opportunities for more closely shared work, particularly around the closure. Devising new assessment models and projects in and out of the hospital are some of the examples illustrated in both Chapter One and this chapter.

The observation of the multidisciplinary core team in operation outside the hospital has demonstrated the tendency of psychiatrists and unit managers to prevent the emergence of a team where the contribution of different disciplines is equally valued, and to reintroduce the hegemony of the medical model into a community service, to the point that the psychologist and one social worker left within the first year, while the other social worker was looking for another post.

Marginalization within the social services

The **marginalization within the social services departments**, expressed frequently and acutely by the teams, came as a surprise to the researcher. While it was related to the crisis which two of the Local Authorities were undergoing, it was even more closely connected to the **style of management** at the Assistant Directors' level. It could also have been related to the low priority given to mental health work in most social services departments, perceived as an area not worthy of investing management input beyond the necessary minimum.

Dually marginalized and demoralized workers are hardly in the position to innovate. In fact, of the three groups, morale was higher in the team where every member participated in closure work, and where the channels of communication with the Assistant Director were considerably more mutual and freer, highlighting two of the necessary conditions for successful innovation. The more satisfactory state of affairs in this department at the time of study demonstrates that the style of management is not so much a structure given, but depends more on personal style and departmental culture. Yet even the third team was not forthcoming with innovative suggestions and felt, no less keenly, the marginality within the hospital. In fact, that team has decided recently (May 1990) to pull out from closure work, partly due to the difficulties experienced in interdisciplinary work and partly to being excluded from the newly formed teams in the community.

A sense of doom and helplessness

A third factor likely to dampen readiness to innovate was the **sense of doom** as to the likelihood that the Government, the Health and Social Services Authorities, would get community services right this time round, and the **helplessness** of the workers who did not feel that they could influence what was happening in any meaningful way beyond the level of the individual client. It was difficult to judge to what extent this perceived helplessness could have been reduced with a more collective stance taken by the teams concerning decisions by the health and social services management, as no such situations have taken place during the study period.

Influencing factors in the wider context

We need to ask ourselves to what extent are social workers prepared for innovation in general, and for closure work in particular, in their qualifying education, in-service training and by working as basic-grade social workers. The answer is not encouraging. The continuing focus in many social-work courses on work with individuals and families is based on working with people who have not been institutionalized, and rarely considers the needs of people with a long institutional history. The lack of sufficient training for group and community work (both of which are as crucial for closure work as for individual work) and the lack of training students to be innovative are some of the striking omissions within the educational process. The current emphasis in social-work agencies on following legislation, administrative regulations, loyalty to the agency first and to the client second, does not encourage workers to innovate. The sad fact that, so far, most of the initiative concerning closure has been left to the Health Authorities adds to the message that closure work is not that important for social workers to engage in.

The threat to the centrality of social work in community mental health relates also to the view of other professionals that social workers' tasks need to be carried out, but not necessarily by social workers. As already mentioned in the introduction to the book, assessment, care management and inspection are going to be the new key functions of any professional or non-professional workforce in mental health services, of which social workers could be one element. It is likely to become attractive in a climate of financial competition for service contracts for a local authority and for a health authority to employ home helps and/or nurses as care managers, as has been already illustrated by Challis and Davies (1986), and Davies and Challis (1986) in relation to work with older clients. Unless social workers are able to demonstrate their ability to offer a **qualitatively** better service they will not be employed in mental health social work. There are considerable training implications resulting from the new requirements; these will be addressed in the conclusion.

The above description highlights some of the challenges that closure work signifies and in which the contribution of social work could be central. It should be remembered that, despite all of the upheaval that local government and social work have been through in the 1980s, social workers have been in the forefront of innovation in mental health work during the same period (Milroy, 1988; Brandon, 1991).

Given the lack of basic information, it is not possible to generalize from the findings of this study to the rest of mental health social work even though there is evidence to suggest that the size of the teams, their structure, the hospital context and the closure process are fairly typical of similar establishments in Britain. Yet it is hoped that the lessons to be learned from this specific experience can be taken further by other teams and departments into the analysis of their own context.

Relevance to other mental health workers

Are the findings of this small-scale study relevant to other mental health professionals? I would argue that the sense of alienation of 'grass-root' workers within the large hospital is not limited to social workers, even though some of the reasons may differ. The exclusion of basic grade workers from the decision-making process concerning closure and the imposition of the decisions made from above are related to initial fears of job losses and, later, to uncertainties as to the changing nature of the professional role, as well as to the lack of adequate preparation for this change at the attitudinal, conceptual and skill-training levels. These are added to the underlying sense that the closure implies a critical view of the work carried out by these workers in the hospital. The scepticism concerning the Government, Health and Social Services readiness and ability to implement the structural change that is necessary is also shared among all mental health workers, even if each group shifts more blame to the 'other place'. None of the professional organizations has so far paid much attention to the psychological and social costs of the closure to the workers, or to the training needs already identified. These training needs too are shared, and are not unique to social workers.

This study has also illustrated that a **participative management style, and ensuring that each worker is directly involved in the challenging aspects of the change process** are useful devices to secure the readiness of workers to invest themselves in this process. Any reader familiar with innovative projects in the field of urban renewal or in private enterprise would have been able to provide us with this practical advice, which is based, in turn, on basic rules of how teams work effectively. It is disconcerting that, for the sake of assumed administrative efficiency, already existing knowledge and expertise has been allowed to be over-looked, rendering the process of closure not only more demoralizing than it need be, but also much less effective than it could have been.

SUMMARY

Is there a place for a more positive line of action to be taken by the local teams that find themselves in the midst of a hospital closure? Based on the teams studied, several promising components emerge. For example, the three teams could and should work out together a training programme that would provide more knowledge and skills in closure work, work in new settings in the community, the development of users' involvement and normalization, innovation and care management. Members of the teams can actively contribute from their own experience to such a training programme. The solidarity that the three teams can share may support them in the inevitable conflicts with the hospital management and/or other disciplines.

They would also need to develop further areas of work that clearly combine work in the hospital with work in the community. For example, one person from the teams was active in establishing a relatives' group in the community, which she ran together with a social worker from an area team. With the hospital about to close, workers should attempt to work part of the time in community mental health facilities outside, such as those being currently developed as part of the specific British Mental Health Grants Scheme.

While it would be desirable to have also equal commitment from the top (i.e. a 'top-to-bottom' approach) together with a 'bottom-up' initiative, there is no need for workers to wait for it to happen and do nothing about the challenges facing them in the meantime. In the meantime, workers can attempt to develop their own ideas, within their realm of professional freedom, however relative that realm may be.

This chapter has focused on the identification of the major issues that hospital closure confronts professional workers with. It has also attempted to delineate the knowledge and skills that are required for closure work.

REFERENCES

Allen, P., Pahl, J. and Quine, L. (1990) *Care Staff in Transition.* HMSO, London.
Austin, R. and Hershey, W. (eds) (1982) *Handbook of Mental Health Administration.* Jossey Bass, San Francisco.
Bachrach, L. (1983) Concepts and issues in de-institutionalization. In: Brofsky, I., Hudson, R. (eds) *The Chronic Psychiatric Patient in the Community.* MTP Press, Lancaster.
Barker, I. (1989) *Multidisciplinary Teamwork.* Central Council of Education and Training in Social Work, London.
Barker, I. and Peck, E. (eds) (1987) *Power in Strange Places.* Good Practices in Mental Health, London.
Basaglia, F. (ed.) (1968) *L'Istituzine Negata.* Einuadi, Roma.
Battaglia, G. (1987) The expanding role of the nurse and the contracting role of the hospital in Italy, *International Journal of Social Psychiatry,* **33**, 115–18.
Becker, H. (1967) *The Boys in White.* The Free Press, New York.
Brandon, D. (1989) *The Trick of Being Ordinary.* Good Impressions, London.
Brandon, D. (1991) *Innovation without Change?* Macmillan, London.
Brearly, P. (1972) *Risk in Social Work.* Routledge, London.
Brooker, C. (1990) (ed.) *Community Psychiatric Nursing, A Research Perspective.* Chapman & Hall, London.
Brown, P. (1985) *The Transfer of Care.* Routledge, London
Burti, L. and Mosher, L. (1989) *Community Mental Health: Principles and Practice.* Norton, New York.
Carson, J. and Bartlett, H. (1990) *Care in the Community — Are the Staff as Stressed by the Changes as the Patients?* Paper given at the TAPS (Team for the Assessment of Psychiatric Services) Annual Conference, London, July 5th.
Castel, R., Lovell, A. and Castel, F. (1982) *The Psychiatric Society.* Columbia Press, New York.
Challis, D. and Davies, B. (1986) *Case Management in Community Care: An Evaluated Experiment in the Home Care of the Elderly.* University of Kent, Canterbury.
COHSE (1983) *The Future of Psychiatric Services.* Draft Report. Confederation of Health Service Employees, London.
COHSE (1991) *Where's the Care? An Investigation into London's Mental Health Services.* Confederation of Health Service Employees, London.
Cooper, J. E. (1990) Professional obstacles to implementation and diffusion of innovative approaches to mental health care. In: Marks, I. and Scott, R. (eds) *Mental Health Care Delivery: Innovations, Impediments and Implementation.* Cambridge University Press, Cambridge.
Crepet, P. (1983) Psychiatry without asylums: origins and prospects in Italy, *International Journal of Health Services,* **13**, 119–129.
Davies, B. and Challis, D. (1986) *Matching Resources to Needs in Community Care: An evaluated demonstration of a long-term care model.* Gower, London.

Del Guidice, G. (1991) How can Mental Hospitals be Phased out? In: Ramon, S. (ed.) *Psychiatry in Transition*. Pluto Press, London.

De Nicola, P. (1991) Changing Professional Roles in the Italian Psychiatric System. In: S. Ramon, (ed.) *Psychiatry in Transition*. Pluto Press, London.

England, H. (1986) *Social Work as Art*. Allen and Unwin, London.

Etzioni, A. (ed.) (1969) *The Semi-professions and Their Organization*. The Free Press, New York.

Friedson, E. (1970) *Professional Dominance*, Atherton, New York.

Froland, D. L. (1981) *Helping Networks and Human Services*. Sage, London, p. 57–59.

Glynn, A. (1991) User participation in a housing project. Innovation Project Report, Diploma in Mental Health Work, London School of Economics, London.

Harlin, C. (1987) Community care in West Germany: Concept and reality. *International Journal of Social Psychiatry*, **33 (2)**, 105–10.

Health and Personal Social Services Statistics (1991). HMSO, London.

Illich, I. (1968) *The Disabling Professions*. Marion Boyars, London.

Ingleby, D. (1981) Understanding mental illness. In: Ingleby, D. (ed.) *Critical Psychiatry*. Penguin, Harmondsworth.

Johnson, T. (1973) *Professions and Powers*. Macmillan, London.

King, D. (1991) Replacing mental hospitals with better services. In: Ramon, S. (ed.) *Psychiatry in Transition*. Pluto Press, London.

Lamb, R. (1990) Will we save the homeless mentally ill? *American Journal of Psychiatry*, **147**, 649–651.

Menzies-Lyth, I. (1988) *Containing Anxiety in Institutions*. Free Associations, London.

Miller, P. and Rose, M. (1986) (eds) *The Power of Psychiatry*. Polity Press, Oxford.

Milroy, A. (1988) Mutual help groups in mental health, *Social Work Today*, 14–16.

Milroy, A. and Hennelly, R. (1989) Changing our professional ways. In: A. Brackx, and Grimshaw, C. (eds) *Mental Health Care in Crisis*. Pluto Press, London.

Nottingham Patients Councils Support Group (NGA) (1989) *Patients' Councils Information Pack*, Nottingham Advocacy Alliance, Nottingham.

Ovretviet, J. (1986) *The Organization of Multidisiciplinary Community Teams*. Health Service Centre, Brunel.

Parry, N. and Parry, J. (1976) *The Rise of the Medical Profession*. Croom Helm, London.

Patmore, C. (1987) *Life After Mental Illness*. Croom Helm, London.

Payne, R. (1987) *Stress in Health Professions*. Wiley, Chichester.

Pirella, A. (ed.) (1982) *I. Tetti Rossi* Provincia di Arezzo.

Pirella, A. (1987) The Implementation of the Italian psychiatric reform in a large conurbation, *International Journal of Social Psychiatry*, **33(1)**, 119–31.

Ramon, S. (1983) Psichiatria democratica: A case study of an Italian community mental health service, *International Journal of Health Services*, **13**, 307–24.

Ramon, S. (1985a) *Psychiatry in Britain: Meaning and Policy*. Croom Helm, London.

Ramon, S. (1985b) Out in the cold in the sunshine state: De-institutionalization in California, *Community Care*, May 9th, 15–17.

Ramon, S. (1985c) The Italian psychiatric reform. In: Mangen, S. (ed.) *Mental Health in the European Community*. Croom Helm, London.

Ramon, S. (1989) The reactions of English-speaking professionals to the Italian psychiatric reform, *International Journal of Social Psychiatry*, **35 (1)**, 120–8.

Ramon, S. (1990) The relevance of symbolic interaction perspectives to the conceptual and practice construction of leaving a psychiatric hospital, *Social Work and Social Sciences Review*, **1 (3)**, 163–76.

Sain, F., Norcio, B. and Malannino, S. (1990) Compulsory health treatment: The experience of Trieste from 1978 to 1988, *For Mental Health*, **14**, 137–52.

Salzberger-Wittenberg, I. (1978) *A Kleinian Approach to Social Work*. Routledge, London.

Satyamurti, C. (1982) *Occupational Survival*. Blackwell, London.

Sheppard, M. (1991) Social work and community psychiatric nursing. In: Abbot, P. and Wallace, C. (eds) *The Sociology of the Caring Professions*. Falmer Press, Brighton.

Smith, G. and Cantley, C. (1985) *Assessing Health Care: A Study in Organizational Evaluation*. Open University, Milton Keynes.

Test, M. A. and Stein, L. (eds.) (1978) *Alternatives to Mental Hospital Treatment*. Plenum, New York.

Tomlinson, D. (1991) *Utopia, Community Care and the Retreat from the Asylum*. Open University Press, Milton Keynes.

Toren, N. (1972) *Social Work as a Semi-profession*. The Free Press, New York.

Tranchina, P. and Basaglia, F. (eds) (1979) *Un Autobiografia di'un Movimento*. p. 1–9. Unione Province Italiane, Regione Toscana, Amminstrazione Provinciale di Arezzo.

Vasconcelos, E. (1991) *Alienists of the Poor: The Development of Community Mental Health in Bel Horizonte, Brazil*. London, PhD Thesis, the London School of Economics.

Warner, R. (1991) Building programmes. In: S. Ramon (ed.) *Beyond Community Care: Normalization and Integration work*, Mind/ Macmillan, London.

White, E. (1990) Surveying CPNs, *Nursing Times*, **86 (51)**, 62–8.

4

The experience and perspectives of patients and care staff of the transition from hospital to community-based care

CHRISTINE PERRING

INTRODUCTION

About this section

This section is based on research into the experience of hospital closure from the patients' perspective. It focuses on the connections between theory, policy and their practical effects at the grassroots level. The study followed three groups of patients through the process of leaving hospital and settling into group homes in the community. It was approached from an anthropological perspective, which relies on participant observation methods and attempts to explore and understand the world view of the subjects of research. Hence, the main interest is in the life experiences of the former patients, how these are interpreted and how they are related to the structures surrounding them.

The group homes, which I will describe in the sections to follow, are modelled in opposition to the image of psychiatric hospitals — large, impersonal and segregated dwellings — an image that has been drawn from much sociological work since the 1950s. The group homes aim to create a different structure and ethos from the hospital, to provide rehabilitation and to break down institutionalism. They are modelled on various ideas of care, but use notions of kinship for a guiding philosophy. They are intended to be domestic in scale and character — 'an ordinary house in an ordinary street'. Despite this, they remain inward-looking: little attention has been given in the reprovision programme to social re-integration and changing attitudes within the family, the neighbourhood or the wider society. The asylums themselves were initially described as model institutions, so we need to ask how far the new 'model institutions' may be influenced by the caring and controlling functions of the asylums.

Will they inherit these functions in a basically continuing form, or will the move to the community change the roles and nature of the mental health services?

This account of the move to community-based care for long-stay patients and care staff explores the way tensions, such as those between caring and controlling, may persist in the shift from one social institution to another. It suggests that, without careful and sensitive work on the principles and practicalities of service provision, institutional forms are likely to be reproduced. Working for change is never simple, as the accounts in this book have shown, but there are positive areas to be worked on. Important among these are the positive responses of many long-stay patients to a situation that is new and insecure, and the commitment of care staff, on which new working practices can be built.

My expectation was that change would be considerable and in many ways this was confirmed. Life outside hospital was preferred by all but a few of the former patients involved, who remained ambivalent and unsure about the changes they experienced. Group home residents spoke positively of the changes in their living environment. They described the pleasures of living in a house with their own rooms, with relatively ordinary facilities and some new choices in their lifestyles and activities. However, their accounts and my own observations show that these changes occurred in a limited and relative way. Residents felt that important aspects of their experience and identities were framed in much the same way they had been as hospital patients.

Research and its theoretical basis

Anthropology

The research was conducted within an anthropological framework, relying mainly on participant observation as well as analysis of documents. The main advantage of this approach is that it allows the researcher to form a picture of what a social institution or event is like for the participants. The aim is to understand the insider's viewpoint, as well as to take a more distanced and analytical view. Official statements of reality — in interviews, policy documents and so on — can be compared with what participants say and do in everyday situations. One of my main aims has been to bring out the patients' perspectives. By describing and reflecting on their histories, their current and changing lives, they were able to show the coherence and validity of such a viewpoint.

Exploring a number of viewpoints has theoretical as well as methodological significance — particularly in showing how a picture of reality is constructed, rather than something that is simply there to be discovered as objective fact. The 'world view' of different participants in a social system is influenced by the cultural construction of meaning and the lived experience of different social groups. (Bourdieu, 1972). Conflict between different groups can be understood as an outcome of differing interests, influenced by differing values and perspectives on their experiences.

This account takes what is essentially an interpretive approach, based upon the view that relations between means and ends are complex and cannot be isolated in the way that positivist social science aims to do. It also takes a dialectical approach, in examining the contradictions that arise in social and historical situations, and in setting different versions of reality alongside each other. This follows the lines of critical medical anthropology, which aims to analyse medicine as a cultural system (Kleinman, 1980). This rationale views an institution to be culturally and historically specific, and does not assume the objectivity or universality of the dominant way of understanding the world (Kuhn, 1970). Despite the idea that because they are segregated, they are outside of society, such institutions cannot be analysed as something apart. Their forms are influenced by wider structures, attitudes and social relations.

In anthropological writing, culture is often described as 'a web of meaning' (Evans-Pritchard, 1937; Geertz, 1973). This view of culture is not a static one, however, where meaning is (as it often appears within a certain culture) unchanging and unchangeable. Institutions are culturally framed and socially constructed, and so come to take on an authority that leads individual members to experience them as a 'datum' or something that is given and taken as fact (Menzies-Lyth, 1970). Individuals are continually reproducing such 'data' as part of the social order, yet altering them as part of lived experience. Douglas (1987) writes about institutions in this broad sense and focuses on the significance of 'the thought world' on the nature of social institutions. In a similar way, Bourdieu's concept of 'habitus' (1972) brings out the significance of social history to understanding present day structures of thought and action. Douglas argues that:

> *'to acquire legitimacy, every kind of institution needs a formula that founds it rightness in reason and in nature...past experience is encapsulated in an institution's rules so that it acts as a guide to what to expect from the future. The more fully the institutions encode expectations, the more they put uncertainty under control, with the further effect that behaviour tends to conform to the institutional matrix.'*

> *(Douglas, 1974, pp. 45, 48).*

Since reality is usually presented from the viewpoints of those who are more powerful, there is a need for research to concentrate on the viewpoints of those whose voices have rarely been heard.

A social role?

In this framework, illness is viewed as a social role: the concept of disease refers to biological reality, illness to social reality, that is the experience of being ill. It is in this sense that I use the term mental illness. This thinking rests on the patterns of recognizing and responding to illness, which have such an important impact on peoples' lives, as well as being influenced by those lives (Taussig, 1980; Dingwall, 1976). The concept of the sick role was first outlined by Parsons (1951) and provided a means of understanding illness in this way.

Box 4.1   Parsons' sick role theory: The sick role legitimates removal of normal social roles and obligations, in return for an obligation to co-operate with the healer, to seek to get well and return to normal roles. This was seen by Parsons as an 'ideal type' but it is a model that applies more readily to acute rather than chronic illness. It does not really address the possibility of conflict between the interests of the sick person and the healer or of the way in which mental illness is generally defined and the emphasis on normal social roles. Mental illness is defined in terms of deviation from such roles, yet the ill person is required to accept his sick state in order to be seen as normal.

Critiques of psychiatric institutions have arisen largely from sociological theory, but often drawing on ethnographic research principles. They have also come from social history (Scull, 1977; Foucault, 1967; Skultans, 1979; Busfield, 1986) and from critical psychiatrists such as Barton and Maxwell-Jones (and more recently, for example R.D. Scott in the UK and Basaglia in Italy). Whereas, in Italy, (Basaglia, 1982) critical psychiatry has been associated with wider political reform movements (Ramon and Giannichedda, 1988), see Chapter Three in this book), in the UK and the USA much of this work has been apolitical and limited, on the whole, to looking at the internal structure of asylums (Goffman, 1968a; Perrucci, 1974).

Critics have also drawn strongly on deviancy and labelling theory in social science, which have been described in the Introduction to this book. A particularly clear account of the impact of labelling in mental health services was provided by Rosenhan's (1973) pseudo-patient study.

Box 4.2   Rosenhan's article 'On being sane in insane places' recounts how a number of volunteers presented themselves to psychiatric hospitals as hearing voices, under instruction to behave normally once admitted. Only fellow patients doubted their madness. They were discharged after a period averaging several weeks, with the diagnosis unquestioned and were categorized as 'in remission'.

This study confirms and contributes to labelling theory, firstly through analysing the way in which assessment and selection of patients for community facilities is carried out and secondly, the attitudes and actions of community staff towards their residents. In particular, the ways in which problems are defined and resolved reveals something of the ways in which labelling operates in care practice.

Institutionalism

Critiques of psychiatric institutions have centred particularly on the concept of institutionalism. The work of Barton, who coined the term 'institutional neurosis', had a significant impact on thinking about psychiatry in the 1950s.

Box 4.3   In his *Institutional Neurosis* Barton (1959) argued that institutional life itself could be seen to account for much of the behaviour in asylums which had been categorized as symptoms of mental illness. It outlined key features of the environment that could contribute to such a condition and described typical effects such as passivity, stooped posture and shambling. He also made it clear that staff/patient relations in such situations could not be ignored and that bullying of various forms was inherent in many regimes.

This work highlighted the problems of separating illness symptoms and institutional and treatment effects on the individual. Personal history can be seen as important to this, yet even today professionals are reliant on medical case histories. As reductive accounts, which reduce the history of the person to signs and symptoms of pathology (Ingleby, 1981) these are inadequate for the work now taking place in the transition from hospital to community.

> 'The patient is pinned down to a few cut-and-dried epithets, with no hint of the complex ambiguities of human conduct or the context in which the patient acts or is observed.'
>
> (Ingleby, 1981, p. 29).

These ideas were developed further by Goffman's work *Asylums* (1968), which introduced the notion of the patient's moral career, and also his work on the presentation of self (1971) and interaction ritual (1967). His work on 'total institutions' focused on the internal structure and routines of asylums and comparable institutions. His account (which could be described as phenomenological) showed how the removal of normal patterns of activity, and means of identity, framed the social life of the asylum.

> **Box 4.4** The features of a 'total institution' are summarized by Goffman (1968, p. 17) as follows:
> 1. All aspects of life are conducted in the same place under the same authority;
> 2. Each phase of daily activity is carried on in the immediate company of others, treated alike and required to do the same thing together;
> 3. All phases are tightly scheduled and imposed from above; and
> 4. There is a basic split between inmates and staff.

What is lacking in this account, however, is a view or a critique of the relationship between the asylum and its wider social context. It is almost as though the idea of the total institution, with its rigid boundaries, placed a boundary on his thinking about the patterns of movement between the asylum and the wider community. The entry to the asylum is analysed, but his view of hospital departure is a very bleak one — the means of transition from the total institution is not explored and little is said about the possibilities for community care.

Since that time, the decreasing length of stay for many patients, with movement in and out of the psychiatric hospital, has altered the nature of such institutions, but in a limited way. Baruch and Treacher's (1978) account of an acute psychiatric unit, for example, highlights the enduring relevance of many ideals on institutionalism. Wing and Brown's (1970) study, moreover, indicates how far the ability of long-term patients to contemplate a life beyond hospital was influenced by lack of a vision of alternatives for them.

Normalization

The principles of normalization are grounded in theories of deviancy and of institutionalism. Wolfensberger's original argument (1972) points to the variation of cultural and social attitudes towards deviancy and suggests that the concept might be regarded as part of a wider (authoritarian) attitude complex. Although this work was grounded in thinking about what was then called mental retardation, his service principles have been taken up and developed more widely (King's Fund, 1980). At their most simple, these principles can be summarized as: (a) an ordinary life; (b) social integration and (c) socially valued roles.

Over time, some problems have emerged with the term 'normalization' and misunderstandings in its application. Wolfensberger stressed that it is not about trying to normalize individuals but about normalizing their conditions of life. Norms for service users were to be understood in the sense of typicality rather than conformity. However, it focused on the social identities of people who had been devalued, and so could be seen as somehow outside of the community, alien or a threat to it, and associated with nature as opposed to culture (Cohen, 1989). Normalization (like hospital closure) could also be seen to represent a challenge to professionalism, to which service providers have experienced difficulty in responding. Since 1981, ideas about normalization have also been confused with the nature of policy shifts towards consumerism in personal social services.

> **Box 4.5** The White Paper *Caring for People* (DOH, 1989) and the Griffiths Report (1988) on community care advocated a principle of consumer choice, based on a range of services, while the Wagner Report 1988 (Sinclair, 1988) on residential care emphasized a principle of positive choice, based on raising the quality and status of caring. *Caring for People*, as the basis for the NHS and Community Care Act 1990 (alongside *Working for Patients*), took up the consumer notion by advocating a 'mixed economy of care'. Nevertheless, the choices advocated in this system are not underpinned by legal rights or advocacy for service users.

The ideals of normalization are reflected to some extent in the policies that I was researching: the way they were put into practice, the focus on everyday life, on homeliness of facilities and so on. While hospital closure itself can be seen as following normalization principles, in terms of scale, location and character of service provision, it is important to examine how far the language or the ideas are carried through into practice. The group home concept — the idea of ordinary homes — appears to exemplify some of this thinking but it was not, in this case, a conscious philosophy so much as one that was felt to be commonsense, natural and caring.

The principles of normalization were also reflected in the research approach: the focus on users' experience, on everyday life, on the life histories and sense of identity of the patients who left; on their wants as opposed to their clinically defined needs.

The policy background

The decision to close these hospitals arose out of a fairly long-standing historical movement but the conceptual and practical bases of the policy have remained unclear. What appears to be a coherent and unified policy involves several strands of thought, which remain quite contradictory.

Far from being an opposition to the medical model of mental illness, historians have stressed that the developments rested on the establishment of a more secure basis for psychiatry within medicine (Busfield, 1986). Social historians such as Jones (1972), who take a progressive and linear view of historical change, have described the philosophy as an outcome of medical development, allowing the return of medical and social care to their proper spheres. The role of the asylums, now called psychiatric hospitals or psychiatric units in general hospitals, would be treatment and rehabilitation rather than care and control. Foucault (1967, p.252), taking a rather different view, described the movement as one of 'madness long since mastered'.

The length of time people spend in hospital has been declining since the mid 1940s due to changes in outlook and therapeutic approaches within institutions as well as the growth of ideas about community care. Throughout the period, the development of community-based mental health services has been very piecemeal. Group homes, therefore, have been around for some time, but the numbers remained small and those that existed were funded largely through benefit-supported rental payments. The quality and level of support services remained low and group homes or hostels were generally not considered for patients who had been in hospital for long periods. Since the late 1970s, the development of such facilities has been aided by joint planning and funding arrangements (Mangen and Rao, 1985) and has been increasingly tied to plans for the closure of the larger Victorian psychiatric hospitals.

So what was the root of the community mental health service plans that followed the decision to close two of the Region's asylums? (See also Chapter 2.) We can outline three strands in the policies that lay behind it. Firstly, there was a movement for integration of psychiatry into more locally based health facilities, concentrating on acute treatment and with long-term care (which psychiatrists are aware has more to do with social care than treatment) being returned to the social domain. Secondly, there was a political movement for redrawing the boundaries of public services into a more private sphere of social care, resting on ideas of individualism and independence, rather than communal responsibility or reciprocity. Thirdly, there was a critical social argument for the integration of mental health services into a more socialized system of care. This third strand draws on the critiques of institutions that I have discussed in the previous section. By examining the experiences of patients and care staff in the hospital closure, we can begin to understand how these policy forces might work through into practice at the ground level and the sorts of conflicts that they reflect.

Community-based mental health services

The factor that distinguishes this closure programme from a more general run-down of hospital beds or a rather slow and piecemeal development of community mental health services, following the 1959 Mental Health Act (Ramon, 1985), is that a decision was made at the Regional Health Authority level to close two hospitals within a planned timetable. This decision was based on a combination of quality and cost factors, since the two hospitals chosen were assessed as providing relatively poor services while having the highest unit costs in the region (NETRHA 1982; c.f Korman and Glennerster, 1985; 1990). The decision was likely to have been influenced also by a series of press scandals about care in one hospital. Although supported by local Community Health Councils and voluntary organizations, it is significant that hospital staff at all levels played little part in the plan.

The hospitals' services were to be replaced by Community Mental Health Services, popularly known as 'reprovision facilities' amongst planning staff, which would completely reprovide the service of the hospital. The broad picture envisaged was of a psychiatric inpatient service centred on the District General Hospital, an outpatient service centred on Community Mental Health Centres and a network of residential and day-care facilities. Early efforts concentrated particularly on the planning of these residential projects — there would have to be a residential placement for each long-stay patient before the hospital could close. Day services were felt by professionals to be important but they lagged behind residential facilities in the planning process, presumably due to the greater urgency given to somewhere to live.

Although strategic planning in each District began in 1983, much of early residential development was opportunistic. Voluntary organizations with a tradition of providing community-based homes, or a concern about the nature of the new facilities came forward to offer a role in the reprovision (McLaughlin, 1990). They also drew in wider sources of finance, such as Housing Association grants, and were able to reduce costs to the Health Authorities by charging residential fees, which could be supported by (then) DHSS benefits.

The resulting pattern was that much of the supported housing available for long-stay patients was designed and managed by voluntary agencies, each with somewhat different philosophies of care. Since this study examines the work of one agency, it is important to realize that the model of care followed here was not the only possible one. While it is, in many ways, typical of organizations providing residential care (c.f. Willcocks *et al.* (1987) on local authority care for elderly people) it is not the only model available.

On the whole, voluntary organizations have specialized in providing small hostels or group homes for residents with long-term needs but not those with the greatest need for support. Following the traditional lines of distinction between health and social care and between statutory and voluntary spheres, health authorities have retained the management of housing for people said to have the highest dependency, with need for nursing care.

In the districts involved in my study, all the residential projects, except those that remained hospital based[1], have followed to some degree principles that could be related to normalization philosophy. They have centred particularly on ideals of 'homeliness' and 'ordinariness' (such as those contained in the more recent recommendations of the Wagner Report (Sinclair, 1988) and the 'Home Life' principles set out by the Social Services Inspectorate (SSI) for residential care for elderly people). The detailed way in which such principles are interpreted and implemented vary, however, in different settings and this is reflected in the differing plans for reprovision facilities.

Elements of the community care philosophy

Recent policy writings around hospital closure and community care have made heavy use of the terms 'community' and 'care' in particular, which are often not clearly defined or explained. It is worth examining the range of meanings attached and the way in which they are used.

The word **community** raises problems due to its vague but all-encompassing associations, which always have a positive symbolic value. I would suggest that some of the problems in use of the community concept (Abrams *et al.*, 1986; Bulmer, 1986) arise from a somewhat over-idealistic image that is so prevalent in British culture. Banton and colleagues (1985) describe this as the 'remembered community' — a notion that is characterized by small scale, boundedness, connectedness and a sense of belonging. They comment that sociologists have tended to apply such a model to the working class, playing down the significance of conflict and power differentials in their lives.

This sort of notion has affected the models of community care that are in operation in this particular hospital closure programme. They are likewise models of a bounded community, drawing on ideas of kinship and connectedness, but they also present the ideal of an alternative community — an exclusively psychiatric one — which is not unlike the original model of the asylums in the 19th century. While the key model for these group homes — that of family care — is inward-looking and is seen in rather idealized terms, the significance of power differentials, such as gender and generational differences, goes unrecognized (Perelberg, 1985).

The ideal notion of community is what Bulmer (1987) describes as 'community lost' in sociological writing. He prefers the notion of 'community regained' which may be based on locality or interest group (Willmot, 1986)

---

[1] One District Health Authority planned to build a new service complex — euphemistically named the Haven — on part of the hospital site. This was to include a medium secure unit for the region, an industrial therapy unit and residential facilities intended for those patients unwilling or unable to move away. Places were to be available to all districts but the other district on which this study was focused opted not to use any of these.

and which is more characteristic of modern urban society where connections are more dispersed, loose-knit and partial. Such a view bears more relation to the context of these hospital closures, where patients are returning, often after many years, to urban neighbourhoods, where ties with former family and friends are often lost and where other routes to social contact may be needed. (For a contrasting context see Towell and Kingsley on the closure of Exeter hospital in Ramon and Giannichedda (1988).)

In policy terms, community may mean much less than this. It simply refers to the provision of services away from a central base (such as the psychiatric hospital) and in smaller-scale units dispersed throughout the district. As suggested in the footnote on page 131, the situation is not quite this clear-cut. Although most services fit this pattern, acute services and some psychogeriatric services are still provided at the district general hospital. Most housing **is** in small local units, but some homes are grouped on one site. The scale of new homes varies from single accommodation to homes for more than ten people sharing, with most somewhere between the two.

The term **care**, like community, is loaded with positive symbolic associations. The provision of care tends to be opposed to **cure** as something natural and intuitive and this view has been important in the way understandings of community-care have developed. Caring is seen as a definitively female role and, despite the attribution of naturalness and positive symbolism surrounding this, the status given to those who give or receive care is generally low (Stacey, 1988; Lewin and Olesen, 1985). So, our ideas of care are culturally defined, relying particularly on gender and kinship values.

Caring also raises the issue of responsibility: whether this is an individual or communal matter, and whether community-care policy refers to care 'in' or care 'by' the community (Walker, 1982; Finch and Groves, 1983). We shall see, in the section on the selection and preparation of patients to leave hospital, that dependency is a basic category, a sort of counterpart to care, which is used by staff to think about how patients fit within the psychiatric system and in the wider society.

THE PSYCHIATRIC HOSPITAL: FROM SOCIOLOGICAL CRITIQUES TO THE
PATIENTS' VIEWPOINTS

Although much has changed in hospital practice since Goffman's account of the 'total institution' (see Box 4.4), certain basic features of Goffman's model are still significant. This is best illustrated by a summary of the features of ward life as observed and described to me by former patients. The ward is as seen by patients as having:

1. A rigid and childlike routine that is ordered by staff roles;
2. A conduct of life on a large-group scale;
3. A lack of privacy;
4. A lack of choice;
5. Barriers to ordinary activity, leading to loss of living skills;
6. Ordinary activity re-categorized as therapy and rehabilitation;
7. Distant staff/patient relations;
8. Patients that are treated as objects, rather than individuals;
9. Patients that are continually observed, yet not known;
10. Heavy reliance on medication as a main form of treatment and control;
11. An apparent, structurally defined inability to do the right thing.

The accounts given to me by patients echo the writing of Goffman and later writers on the nature of institutionalism (Perrucci, 1974; Baruch and Treacher, 1978). Residents' accounts confirmed the relevance of such work today. Jane said that:

> '... patients were always referred to as 'them' not people. The nurses generally sit in their office, come out to do a few things, then go back in again, thinking they've done a lot of work. They talk to each other rather than to patients on the whole.'

Box 4.6 Daily timetable for the ward which three group home residents left:

7 a.m.   Day shift begins, domestic tasks on the ward for some patients;

8 a.m.   Breakfast on the ward;

9 a.m.   Workshops or other structured activity[a], frail patients and a few others remain on the ward;

11 a.m.   Coffee break in workshops;

12 a.m.   Lunch on the ward;

2 p.m.   Return to the workshops;

3 p.m.   Tea break in the workshops;

4 p.m.   Return to ward for tea (last meal of the day);

7 p.m.   Occasionally bingo, or attend a social on one ward;

9.30–10 p.m.   Official bedtime. Hot drinks before bed with medication. Medication dispensed from a trolley at set times, related to meal times.

[a]Some patients did not attend workshops, due to frailty or personal decision not to do so, but the latter choice was not easily accepted by staff. Residents also described how 'a good nurse' might be more flexible over bedtimes and allow you to sit with them and watch the late film.

Maurice explained that in hospital you didn't get enough help for various reasons — the attitude of the nurses and there not being enough of them. He said that they stay in the office most of the time and do not talk to people very much. The patients tend to be thrown together. He remarked that the nurses do not help people in the way that they need, if at all; and that they didn't help him in the way that he needed.

The nature of the ward as experienced by patients is defined to a significant degree by the structure of the hospital: not only its architectural form (Foucault, 1979) but by its pyramidal working structure (Fig. 4.1). This hierarchy operates with small numbers of high-level staff and increasing staff-patient ratios and contact towards the base of the pyramid — the patients themselves.

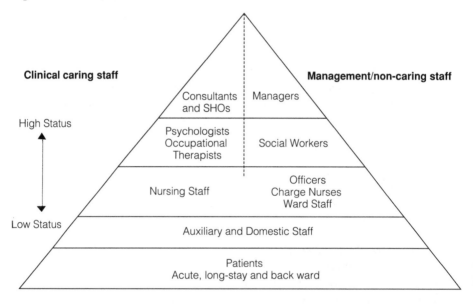

Figure 4.1   The hospital pyramid.

Lack of direct patient contact

Lack of direct patient contact in this system becomes a marker of status: those with the most formal power have little role in care. This pattern relates to the basic gender and class divisions instituted in hospitals generally with a triad of doctor, nurse and patient, seen metaphorically as paternal, maternal and childlike in roles. The account of group home life will show how such a pattern has been carried into service structures outside the hospital.

There is also a secondary and cross-cutting distinction between professional groups, which relates to the basic division of clinical and social/

psychological models of medicine. The first line of division is between clinical and managerial staff (instituted by the 1984 general management system for the health service) which is described by nurses as 'caring' and 'non-caring' staff. The second division lies between medical and paramedical or social services staff which basically differentiates nurses and doctors from psychologists, occupational therapists and social workers.

Lack of privacy

One of the over-riding features of the ward environment, beyond the imposed routine, was the lack of privacy the patients experienced, framed by the design of the ward itself, but also by its running. The dormitory was the general sleeping area and the use of cupboards and curtains for screening had little effect visually or in terms of sound. Such an arrangement does little for individual self-esteem in a society with clear and high regard for personal privacy.

As a result, patterns of sleeping and of day-time activity could be disturbed. Two residents described to me how they had become dependent on sleeping tablets, prescribed when they were disturbed by a restless patient. The staff response had not been to rethink the nature of the environment but to react to the symptoms. In this way, an external source of trouble became their own, internalized sleep problem. The television, which was switched on constantly throughout the day at a volume to accommodate the hard of hearing, was extremely disruptive to discussion groups on the ward, yet no one felt able to turn it off. It was complained about within the discussion group but accepted. In this, one can see that the need to become accepting and to relinquish choice can become a part of learning to fit to the institutional environment.

Lack of choice

Choice, for patients, was limited in many small ways that most individuals would take for granted, yet those residents who did not fit told me that they had found that, living in this situation, they were required to be passive in order to be viewed as normal.

Jane said she still could not understand why they designed the hospitals as they were. 'Why don't they allow people to continue doing things like cooking their own food instead of the awful stuff, slops, which they provide?' The staff had told her that many patients could not do that. She felt they should have smaller places. On another occasion, she explained that one of the reasons why she was so set against day centres was her experience in hospital of being pressurized to do 'IT' (industrial therapy) rather than painting.

Mary commented on how much more responsibility there was outside '... in hospital it's all taken off you'. She finds it quite hard after such a long time, she explained, to manage responsibility for her own life, but she liked the greater scope. 'In hospital they work you physically, but not the mind. My mind's always been no good though.'

Lack of facilities

A further feature contributing to the institutionalism spoken about by nurses and community-based staff was the lack of facilities to assist patients in acting or caring for themselves. Meals were provided, at set times and with little choice, by a central kitchen. On many long-stay wards, not even facilities for making tea and snacks, or for doing laundry, were available to patients. One nurse, for example, described to me a curious set of rules by which patients on his wards were prevented from boiling a kettle or obtaining hot water to make tea. He explained to me that he **was** keen to try and help with preparation for living outside hospital but what could he do when he wasn't even allowed to use a spare phone for the men to practise making phone calls?

Domestic work was undertaken by patients on a ward scale, rather than centring on care of personal space or belongings. In some wards, few facilities existed even for the care and safe-keeping of personal property. Several residents explained to me that their lack of good clothing was down to experience of theft as well as sheer lack of money: George's good coat had been stolen and he could not replace it. He made the point that it was simply not worth saving up for good 'stuff' in hospital.

The implications of the ward environment for rehabilitation are considerable. It is one that not only leads to loss of skills, but to loss of motivation to care for oneself. Even though, for the long-stay patients, it is primarily a place of residence rather than treatment, the hospital is managed around the principle of controlling or containing sickness. The regulation of time, through the ward routines, the medication round and so on, is one element in the loss of self-direction that the patients experienced. Routines could be said to have a therapeutic function, in enabling people to feel a certain sense of security in the regularity of their lives. However, in the rigid routine of the ward system, the regulation is removed and imposed from above in a way that fails to prepare patients for life outside.

Preparation of patients to leave hospital

It is in this light that there is very little to say about the preparation of patients in hospital for leaving. Much of the work was done by staff who were not ward-based. Those nursing staff who supported or at least accepted the closure policy, expressed frustration at the lack of facilities or training to assist them in rehabilitation, and confusion over the changes in priority that were being advocated by administrators. Those who felt some hostility to or anxiety about the closure declined to co-operate with arrangements made for preparation, or attempted to sabotage work by mixing up arrangements and 'talking patients down'. At the same time, project-based staff were attempting to open up interest and discussion about living outside the hospital.

Patients, therefore, received mixed messages about preparation for leaving, in a context that was intrinsically discouraging. It should hardly surprise us that a group of people who felt threatened in terms of professional self-esteem and job security and who lacked confidence would not be in a good position to prepare patients for leaving. In practice, staff for early housing projects worked largely without active participation from hospital staff. Could there have been another way? Since the time of this study, arrangements for training of nursing staff have been set in motion, with the aim of preparing them for working in different ways.

It appears that to carry nurses along, as participants in the process rather than those left behind, certain policy directions would have been helpful. Firstly, an assurance about job security, re-deployment and training early in the process may have helped to reassure ambivalent staff and prepare **them** for the future. Secondly, training would need to be focused on working in closer personal co-operation **with** (rather than for) patients and in the necessary communication skills. Thirdly, this would need to be under-pinned by a democratization of hospital structures.

Box 4.7 A possible model for re-orientation for hospital staff? Rotelli (in Ramon and Giannichedda, 1988, p.183) describes how, before the closure of the asylum in Trieste began, wards began to work in a different way. The principle was that the institution should change from within in order to ensure sustainable change that would translate into the development of services in the community.

Models for staff training are available in the UK, which could be used by hospital and community-based staff. These are oriented mainly around gaining insight into the patients' experience and building on this to help to prepare them for change, for example:

1. *What Matters Most*: a training pack providing exercises for staff to put themselves in the users' shoes.
2. *Getting to Know You*: a means of assessing or working with patients, based on life history and one to one contacts.
3. *PASS*: a training and service evaluation exercise, centred on normal-ization principles.

Why not try one of these approaches in your college or workplace? Details are given at the end of this chapter.

SELECTION AND PREPARATION OF PATIENTS TO LEAVE HOSPITAL

This section explores the way in which selection and preparation was developed through practical experience, the way patients and staff responded to wider uncertainties about the closure, and the limitations they placed on the nature of change.

The first stage of the transition process for patients and care staff is breaking the news of closure. As suggested above, the accounts of the transition given to me indicate that this was done in a way that produced ambivalence for staff and patients. Nursing staff had not been involved in the initial plans at regional level. The production of a consultation document in 1982 came after a long period of doubt and speculation about the hospitals' future and the closure decision was actively opposed by a number of high-level staff. Two residents, visiting a group home for the first time, told staff that they did not believe the hospital would close — 'the boss' had told them that it would not, and so they were unsure whether to move or to wait and see what happened. After a year of living in a group home, another resident, even though her bed had been 'closed', was told by nursing staff that she should come back in 'for a rest'. It was in this climate of uncertainty in which the early work on selecting and preparing patients for leaving hospital took place.

Policy for selection and preparation was developed jointly (but not without some conflict, misunderstanding and delays) between managerial and professional staff in the Health Authorities, with input from key Social Service managers and the voluntary agencies managing community-based residential projects. While community-based care staff became actively involved in carrying through the plans formed at management level, nurses' roles were marginal. Even though nursing officers had a role in planning and managing the process, and the work was initially hospital-based, the process itself was moulded by the need of both patients and workers to face these changes by turning towards the world beyond the hospital.

Assessment

The selection of patients for different 'reprovision' facilities was grounded on assessment. At the most basic level, this meant determining numbers of patients for each district and a pattern of service needs. When the closure decision was announced, although total in-patient numbers were known, it was not clear who those patients were, where they came from or what sort of accommodation and care they might need. Lack of such basic information added to the difficulties of the planning process. It was also agreed that individual assessment would be needed to facilitate detailed planning and to match individuals or groups of patients to community-based facilities. An important distinction should be highlighted here: while some professionals saw assessment as a means of fitting patients effectively into projects, others saw the proper aim as being to shape project plans around the assessed needs and preferences of the patients. This account shows how in practice, the first approach was followed in early closure projects.

The approaches to assessment that were adopted could be divided into what are essentially clinically and socially-based frameworks. The former is more commonly used by health professionals and is centred on the functioning of patients in the ward setting, to assess the behavioural and related problems of each patient. It does not seek to understand the patient in relation to his or her personal history or relationship with the ward environment. The socially-based approach shifts attention to the types of needs and problems that are likely to emerge in a community setting, in other words the practical and social skills and resources or difficulties of the person. What also distinguishes the two approaches (which may in practice be combined or used alongside each other) is that the socially-based approach can incorporate the factor of personal choice.

In each case, assessment involved some form of staff report and an interview with the patient. The assessment interview can be used in various ways: as a baseline for strategic and detailed planning; to match patients to different reprovision projects; to test clinical observations of patients or to explore attitudes towards leaving hospital, what each person's preferences or aspirations might be, and what losses or gains in quality of life s/he might experience. The socially-based approach is also able to re-evaluate the distortions in image produced by the reductive clinical histories and observations produced in an institutional environment. If the assessment explores the individual's life history and perspectives on the transition (Brost and Johnson, 1982), it may also provide a basis for each patient to prepare for the move and to achieve a greater subjective quality of life after leaving hospital.

The summary given below, of the assessment made for one patient, brings out this contrast. Patients in one of the hospitals were assessed firstly by means of a schedule by which staff rate each patient's behaviour for deviancy and handicap. These are combined into an overall score for dependency where '0 represents a standard of behaviour acceptable in the community; a score of 144 represents total dependency (Carson, 1988, p. 3). This was supplemented, on the initiative of the new resettlement team, by an approach designed to assess the person's ability to cope outside hospital. This was done through examining case notes and by a personal interview with the patient. The latter was designed mainly to gain an overall impression of the patient but also to find out about the person's views and preferences about leaving hospital.

Case study

Howard's case, summarized here for brevity, illustrates the process. Howard, a 30-year-old man, who had been resident in the hospital since 1980, was assessed (using the Hall and Baker schedule) as 'in the most severe handicap category of long stay', having scored 'average' for 'deviant behaviour' and consequently, 'high' for dependency. The report recommended a high level of care and supervision in terms of daily living. He was subsequently assessed by the community psychiatrist, in collaboration with nursing and group home staff. This assessment noted that his psychiatric diagnosis was unclear and doubtful but that he was probably mentally handicapped and possibly suffering from schizophrenia. Brief notes were made on his psychiatric history but no notes were available on his personal history and no social work reports existed.

The charge nurse present commented briefly on his self care, social skills, daily routine and family contacts. The nurse pointed out that little was known about his domestic and other skills since there was little opportunity to exercise them in hospital. After a short interview, in which Howard showed great enthusiasm for moving to a group home, staff commented on his motivation. A recommendation was made that his living skills needed exploration and further training. Group home staff noted as an advantage that his friend on the ward would probably be moving to the house.

What was striking about this, and other assessments, is the relative absence of any history, beyond the reductive and sometimes plainly inac- curate recordings of case notes. Most of the personal information came from nursing staff, from community-based workers who had run discus- sion groups on the ward and from the interviews. It is also notable that the clinical scoring seemed to bear little relation to the impression formed during preparatory home visits or in the more holistic assessment. The clinical assessment was primarily concerned with measuring deficits in behaviour in the restricted ward environment. It took no account of poss- ibilities for change, or of the personal and social history of the person. The later assessment attempted to do this and to gain a more rounded impres- sion of the person, but was limited in this by the characteristics of hospital records and the social context of the ward.

Howard was selected for the group home, despite his high-dependency score, on the basis of his sociability and motivation for leaving. Community- based workers felt that his lack of skill was unimportant, since they had facilities to assist him with this. Conversely, they were reluctant to consider people who may have had lower scores but who they thought would have difficulty in a shared home environment or who might be viewed as socially unacceptable in some way. To understand how such decisions were formed and debated between different groups we need to look at the way workers categorized patients and what these reveal about their assump- tions regarding mental illness and suitability for community living.

Definition

In practice, one of the main purposes of individual assessments was to match different patients to residential projects. Consequently the definitions used followed the lines of distinction that planners made for project development. The projects themselves were assumed to reflect broad categories of patient need, which was described in terms of dependency. Dependency was used, therefore, as an organizing concept: a term that was felt to sum up the essential qualities of a patient and somehow define his or her nature. It offered a means of defining the nature of the rehabilitation and care offered in the community setting. In this way, the qualities of service could come to be seen as arising from the nature of the people for whom it was said to be designed. It became a symbolic means of ordering and negotiating the transition from one institutional form of care to another. Patients and projects were categorized into three broad groups — high, medium and low dependency — so that a process of matching and selection could take place. The forms of accommodation considered matched these basic categories roughly as follows:

1. Independent flats and unstaffed group homes (short-stay and low-dependency accommodation);
2. Group homes with day-time staff (medium-dependency accommodation);
3. Group homes/hostels with 24-h staff/24-h nursing staff respectively (high-dependency accommodation);
4. Hostel/wards on hospital site (special needs accommodation);

The provisional plans for one district, for example, gave numbers of patients expected to need each of these forms of accommodation, in addition to replacement wards at the District General Hospital for acute care and for psycho-geriatric care. The movement from high to low dependency follows a line of movement from more institutional and segregated to more independent and community-oriented forms of care.

As we have seen, however, the concept of dependency was used to sum up a range of personal attributes, taking in ideas about ability or disability, normality, social acceptability or deviancy. Shared understandings about such categorizations were generally assumed, yet staff concerns differed according to their working bases and outlooks. As a result, staff found it difficult to develop a coherent approach to selection.

These differences were compounded by the fears of the hospital-based staff about their residual roles in a closing institution. Much energy focused on the issue of whether selection was about 'creaming off', leaving nurses to cope with an increasingly difficult and demoralized patient group.[2] While selection by community-based staff cut across clinical categories, they felt that motivation for leaving was crucial. Understandably, they wanted to offer chances to those who were keen to leave. The issue was not simple, however, since many patients only began to show active interest in leaving hospital once they had been given the opportunity to talk about it,

---

[2] This process was paralleled in the staff group itself, since only the more confident nurses applied for community-based posts.

to find out what might be available and to visit supported housing projects (Abrahamson and Bremer 1982; Booth *et al.,* 1990).

Criteria for selection

The criteria of selection operate on explicit and implicit levels. The explicit level is concerned with assessment of needs (and to some extent preferences), while the implicit level is concerned with acceptability in relation to social norms and suitability in relation to particular community facilities. Analysing the ideas used by the different workers involved shows how decision-making often relied on implicit criteria used by the different agencies, but was communicated through explicit criteria. As we have noted, this centres on the concept of dependency, which is assumed to have shared meanings. In this way, disagreements over definitions of need and approaches to care are evaded. While avoiding open conflict, the process failed to explore the variety of assumptions involved, causing confusion and contributing to the structural difficulties of collaboration between differing professional and interest groups.

Case study

The case of Alfred shows how the use of explicit and implicit criteria and the failure of different groups to acknowledge this pattern could produce difficulties in co-operation over the transition process.

Alfred had been placed on the list for one of the group homes by the hospital-based resettlement team. He was very keen to leave hospital and had friends in the area. He did not follow any structured day-time activity and went out of the hospital regularly, and so was viewed as being fairly independent. Alfred visited the home several times and care workers felt he was well motivated and able to contribute to the home. Several problems, such as petty thieving in the past, were noted but it was felt that he had 'come a long way'. When Alfred asked if he could choose his bedroom, group home managers were reluctant to make a decision on the move. They told care staff that he was too difficult, would not attend a day centre and would not fit but these views were not directly aired in multi-disciplinary project meetings.

After some delay, both care staff and resettlement staff grew impatient and angry that he had been allowed to visit the house and become attached, when it was becoming increasingly clear that managers did not consider him suitable for group home living. Their view, which was not expressed but hinted at in meetings, was that he was not suitable since he lacked social acceptability. A minority of local residents had responded negatively to the planning application for this home's conversion.[3] Alfred was scruffy

---

[3] Although several local residents initially opposed the planning application for the home, an equal number wrote in positive support of the project. The opposition was largely defused by giving residents more information on the plans.

and, due to deafness, had a rather loud voice. He liked to go out independently, and was already a regular attender at a drop-in club in the borough but would probably not co-operate with the usual rule of regular day-centre attendance. He was sociable but inclined to scrounge for cigarettes. One could conclude that, in the views of managers, he would be unable to 'maintain face' (Goffman, 1971); that is, that he would not be able to present an acceptably managed image in wider social encounters. It is clear that, for Alfred, all the official criteria of selection were considered less important than the implicit consideration of social conformity.

Rehabilitation

For those providing community-based care, rehabilitation is both an aim and a means of enabling long-stay patients to make this move. Theories of institutionalism have shown how the structure and routines of psychiatric institutions have produced disabling environments, in which patients' initial problems are compounded by the reduction of their identities and living patterns. It is in the context of institutionalism, therefore, that the need for and the difficulties of rehabilitation arise.

In the hospital, occupational therapy and industrial therapy were provided for patients away from the ward itself. The majority of men attended the industrial therapy unit, where they did packaging or assembly work and, in a few cases, learned basic skills such as woodworking. Women were more likely to be engaged in domestic tasks related to the ward itself.This work was seen as 'something to do' and a source of extra money, although several patients complained about the nominally low rates given. When patients were being considered for discharge, they could be sent on short rehabilitation courses, within the hospital, where they practised ordinary living skills such as cooking and were assessed on these.

A nurse's viewpoint

One nurse described her experiences with rehabilitation work in hospital. She had come to visit former patients in a group home (the only nurse who, to my knowledge, had done so) and had explained how concerned she had felt about the prospect of their leaving. She described how she tried to prepare people for leaving on the wards and tried to include rehabilitation as part of general care. Traditionally, they had tried to do such things, she said, like cooking a meal in a small group, with a nice setting and sitting down to eat together. This had been stopped, however, because administrators thought nurses were after free food. Now, she said, they were telling them to do it as part of the rehabilitation programme.

A ward-based discussion group

In a recording of a hospital-based discussion group and a group home visit, the interplay of rehabilitation and the outside is brought out. The marginalization of ordinary living skills in hospital makes it difficult for staff and patients to think of rehabilitation in isolation from the issue of leaving hospital itself. These sessions are oriented towards the group home, which provides some focus for these broader issues and a basis for developing relationships between patients and community-based care staff.

In this session, a group of patients from two long-stay wards were meeting with care staff in what was called an 'activation session' by group home managers. Carol (worker) did most of the talking, since the other group home worker was new to the project. I noticed that she talked mainly to the patients she was already familiar with and especially those who had visited the house. The main focus of the discussion was on the house and the idea of moving out to a home of this sort. First she asked a few people why they thought we were all here together:

Maurice : 'For a meeting.'
Carol   : 'What's the purpose of the meeting?'
David   : 'About moving?'
Carol   : 'Yes, about the house which some of you have been to see.'

She then talked about the hospital closure and looking for alternative homes. She asked what (the initials) CRT meant. Maurice replied 'Community Rehabilitation Trust', and they discussed what rehabilitation might mean — living in a house, learning to do things for yourself, like cooking. She asked those who had visited what they thought. Did they like it? All said yes or just nodded.

A group-home visit as preparation for leaving hospital

Five patients visited with three workers, Carol arriving later after talking to ward staff 'about things'. When I arrived, John (worker) was just going in with Maurice and Ada to the kitchen. We looked around the house to see what other furniture had arrived. Ada sat down in the living room, smiled, and said she liked it. Back in the kitchen they sat down with John to set the new alarm clocks and put batteries in, while I put the kettle on. Ada and Maurice both decided they would like coffee. John said they would go shopping, have some lunch, then dinner later and return to the hospital by about 6 p.m.

In a while, Carol and Maria (workers) arrived with David, George and Raj. Raj was wearing a smart new cap and everyone said it suited him. It was very cold and I noticed that no one except Maurice was really adequately dressed — they had no overcoats, scarfs or gloves. Ada had on a thin dress, popsocks and a jacket. While we were having tea, Carol asked David what were his worries about staying overnight. He said he was worried he would not be able to see his sister, if he came to live in the house. He had explained that she was frail and would find it difficult to get there to see him, since it was further away than the hospital. Carol assured him that they would make sure that it would be OK, offering to go with him until he had worked out the way and to collect her in the car if she wanted to come and see the house. She asked if there was anything else he was bothered about, but he did not say that there was.

After tea and biscuits, John asked everyone what they wanted for lunch but got no response. He made a few suggestions and asked if they liked the idea of these. This brought out more opinions and ideas. With some input, he wrote out a shopping list and we split into two groups, one for the supermarket, one for the vegetable market. At the shops, Maria took care to include Raj and David in finding the items on the list, in deciding how much to get and so on. All the shopping was put into a wheely basket, which George pulled back to the house.

This passage also reveals how far ideas for rehabilitation were based on domestic activity. The group homes provide a context for such activity, which had been lacking in the hospital. Beyond preparation for leaving, and once living in the home, it needed to be much more than this. The account of everyday life in group homes will show that rehabilitation was more than this — it was an attempt to resocialize those were seen to be lacking in normal social skills but it was also limited to domestic activity within the home, in such a way that the initial enthusiasm of staff and residents proved difficult to sustain.

In terms of the hospital closure plans, rehabilitation simply means preparing people to move out of hospital, generally into supported housing, in such a way that they can cope with daily living. There is an aim, implied in some of the plans, of the patient moving (literally, by moving on) to more independent forms of housing. Group homes, being conceived as 'homes for life', reflect a view that such progression for long-stay patients is unlikely to occur, and relatively little interest was shown in needs for more sustained rehabilitation approaches, beyond training for leaving hospital. This widespread lack of confidence in rehabilitation is echoed later in the reticence of those providing care to move beyond the sphere of psychiatry to encourage residents' use of ordinary community facilities.

TRANSITIONS

Change and loss

For the long-term patients, the admission to hospital was a major life event. Its effect on their personal and social identity was such that they were conceived by others as patients rather than as ordinary people. For the majority, family and other relationships had been damaged or destroyed. The hospital had become a home, albeit an unsatisfactory one. Now the hospital was to close, they were faced with leaving home. Sociologists and psychologists have analysed the significance of leaving home as a life crisis

(Brown and Harris, 1978; Murray Parkes, 1971). Marris (1974) describes such changes as loss and draws an analogy with the loss of bereavement. He argues that critical changes can only be coped with if new events are put into a framework that continues to be meaningful for the person under-going them. The role of ritual, in his view, is in providing a culturally sanctioned process of mourning loss, which incorporates the conflicting emotions involved into a meaningful framework.

> *'If we believe the meaning of life can only be defined in the experience of each individual, we cannot at the same time treat that experience as indifferent... Such change implies loss and these losses must be grieved for, unless life is meaningless anyway.'*
>
> *(Marris, 1974, p. 91)*

It follows from this perspective that preparation for leaving hospital is about much more than training for more independent living. This perspect-ive was supported by the desire of patients throughout the move to reflect on their experiences and to feel that the transition was marked in some way. It is also revealed in the ambivalence that they sometimes expressed, with feelings of hope and depression, of heightened expectations and the need to reflect on and accept the past.

Leaving hospital as a rite of passage

The entry into the psychiatric hospital has been described as a rite of passage. In the case of people with 'chronic' illness or disability, the ideal model of the sick role (Box 4.1) is broken into a pattern of seemingly endless removal. Garfinkel (1956) described the entry as a 'ceremony of degrada-tion'. Following on from this, Goffman (1968) describes how the entry and stripping away of the patient's previous social identity and the props of everyday life, initiate this 'moral career':

> *'His self is systematically, if often unintentionally, mortified. He begins some radical shifts in his moral career, a career composed of the progressive changes that occur in the beliefs that he has concerning himself and significant others'.*
>
> *(Goffman, 1968, p. 24)*

Anthropologists have shown how, in a wide range of cultural contexts, life crises are marked out and managed through ritual.

Box 4.8   Rites of passage, as first set out by Van Gennep in 1908, follow three main phases: separation, marginal and incorporation. They accompany life crises in a wide range of cultures. The marginal or liminal (from the Latin word for threshold) phase is often charac-terized by seclusion and ideas of both sacredness and danger (Van Gennep, 1960).

The liminal state expresses and symbolically frames the ambiguities that are generally associated with change. Such ambiguities are often associated with notions of anomaly and consequent notions of dangerous power and vulnerability. Douglas, in *Purity and Danger* (1984), shows how the ambiguity of the liminal state leads to notions of ritual pollution and danger. Such ideas are also found in the attitudes of staff surrounding the closure of the hospital and the patients who are leaving. My observations of leaving days, for three groups of patients, suggested that the nature of departure was influenced primarily by staff avoidance and fears about the transition. Following the theory of 'rites of passage' we might expect that the phase of re-incorporation into changed, but restored, social roles might be surrounded by ritual; a completion of the cycle begun with the rites of entry. However, for long-stay patients, the liminal phase had come to be seen as permanent, an unchanging state, until the hospital closure decision far removed from patients and their carers was taken. A special ceremony to mark the departure perhaps, like those given for graduates or those retiring from work? Several residents, in the months after leaving hospital, expressed disappointments linked to the experience of leave-taking.

Diary notes of leaving day

The following diary passage records the leaving day for three patients moving to a group home.

As the worker, Carol, and I arrived in the minibus, we met Jane walking along and she got in to show us where to go. Carol ended up parking outside a fire escape, which led directly onto the ward and went up through it. There were very few patients around, most having gone to the workshops. Those who remained were sitting in armchairs watching TV. One woman said 'goodbye' to Jane and asked if they would be coming back for a visit. The Sister handed over medication for two weeks and an out-patient appointment card to the worker. All their property was already packed up, each person having a bag and/or case plus one or two bin bags. Jane had things for around the house, a couple of cardboard boxes with pottery and paintings in, plus a carrier bag with some plants.

The departure was very low-key. (I recalled it later as being almost silent, a rather dismal affair.) Most patients were not on the ward anyway and the staff made little fuss. The Sister passed their belongings down the fire escape, calling a domestic worker to help her. The three new residents helped, even though I was there to carry bags. They all ended up standing at the bottom of the fire escape, in the pouring rain. No one went back up and no one went out to say goodbye. There was no final wave. All three were due to re-visit the hospital on Monday, to sort out financial matters and Margaret and Hilda were expecting to return regularly to the workshop. Margaret was taking a week's break to settle in first, but Hilda felt she'd taken up her entitlement with the week off preparing to leave.

Jane told me, in the van, that they had had a drink on the ward the previous night as a sort of farewell 'do'. Carol asked if she was pleased to be leaving and she said Yes and no. Later in the day, she talked about the significance of the move several times, talking about 'starting to rebuild our lives'. She felt she was a bit old now to start again; 20 years younger she would have really gone for it, but she said 'I'm different now, from when I left before'.

Discussion

In the history of the long-stay patients who are now leaving the hospital, the point of passage and the liminal identity that had encapsulated it had become a perpetual state. The apparent 'otherness' of a person who is part of society, yet excluded from it, can be understood in this way. The departure from hospital could be approached as a point of transition, to a changed but restored personal and social identity (Ramon, 1990) or alternatively as a continuation of the point of passage where the identity of the person is still that of the patient.

These sorts of ambiguities were reflected in the approach of care staff to departure and the consequent disappointment felt by some former patients. The move was gradual one, starting with short visits and progressing to stays, then to an initial trial period of residence, during which the resident could return to the hospital.[4] The procedures were helpful in offering a sense of stability, giving patients the opportunity to try out and adapt to new circumstances, but some residents felt that they had not really separated from the hospital in the move. Among residents, the move led to reflection on the past course of their lives, to some anxieties and uncertainties but also to renewed hopes for the future, which staff were not fully equipped to respond to. 'You must remember, we're all 10-year patients...there is so much re-adjustment', Jane said. She was trying to explain the stresses associated with the visiting process 'backwards and forwards' which, she said, made her feel more unsettled. For herself, she would prefer a clear-cut thing, just to move in one go. So many people were telling her different things and giving her conflicting views. She herself could see many points on either side and felt very unsettled about it. Gladys was not keen to go back (to the ward) either, she liked the house, she had stayed there and made up her mind.

Staff responses and resistance to change

It could be argued that staff responses surrounding the departure were merely oversight, a gap compared with the considerable effort that went

---

[4] The resident could be returned by staff at any point, but after the trial period patients would not be able to choose to return. Their beds were officially closed after three months. Additionally, no mechanism had been developed to allow unhappy residents to transfer to another placement in the community. Despite this policy, nurses and community-based staff occasionally tried to tempt or to threaten residents with a return to hospital.

into the initial selection and preparation process. I would argue that it related to insecurities and ambivalance amongst the staff, hospital and community-based, about managing the process of transition. For hospital staff, the moves represented a denial of their professional roles and value. For community-based staff it touched on their own attitudes regarding mental illness and towards taking on responsibility for care. While they were strongly committed to the ideals of caring in the community, they were also encouraged to limit their expectations of rehabilitation, and to emphasize continuity within change. Menzies Lyth's (1970) analysis of hospital nursing practice was described in Chapter Three. Figures 4.2, 4.3 and 4.4 summarize some of the continuities and changes in conditions affecting staff responses to anxiety-provoking situations in different care settings (Figs 4.2–4.4).

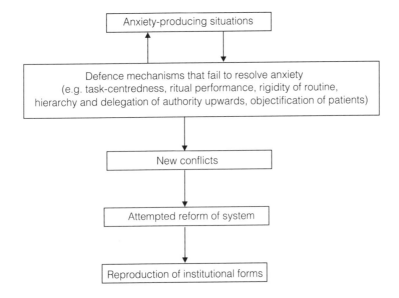

Figure 4.2 Schematic representation of social systems as defences against anxiety in a range of institutional contexts (general hospital, long-stay hospital or residential care).

Following Marris' (1974) argument, we might say that continuity is vital to an individual or cultural capacity to face critical change. In this case, however, it seemed that continuities were related more strongly to organizational and professional demands than to the former patients' personal needs. It could even be seen as failing to respond to workers' personal needs, since both hospital and group-home staff, on the whole, showed

Acute illness/general hospitals	Chronic illness/mental hospitals/residential care
Physical intimacy	Physical intimacy
Patient reliance on nurse (physical and psychological)	Resident reliance on carer (physical and psychological)
Responsibility for treatment	Lack of treatment/cure
Responsibility for life/death	Responsibility for welfare
Fear of death	Fear of madness/disorder
Fear of loss of control	Fear of loss of control

Figure 4.3   Sources of anxiety in various institutional contexts.

Acute illness/general hospitals	Chronic illness/mental hospitals/residential care
Elaborate hierarchy	Shallower hierarchy
Routine–ritual task performance	Routine–balance of rigidity/flexibility
Uniformity of staff as a group	Staff as individuals
Interchangeability not teamwork	Staff isolation
Patients depersonalized and objectified	Residents as individuals but still objectified
Splitting of roles	More holistic roles
Detachment and denial of feelings	Attachment plus detachment and denial of feelings

Figure 4.4   Responses and features in various institutional contexts.

interest in taking on more responsible roles and in opportunities for learning. Marris stresses the importance of the meaningfulness of change and this was clear to me in the desire of former patients to talk about the past in the present, and to make sense of the discontinuities in their lives. Organizational responses to residents' differing reactions to the transition were not so coherent.

Staff responses to two group-home residents
A look at the contrasting staff responses to two residents who had some difficulty in settling into the group home's routine reveals how staff responses were primarily geared to organizational need for order and

certainty. This was not always the case of course. Staff differed in their individual working styles and the degree to which they adapted to such an organizational culture. In many cases, their initial responses could be quite different and revealed a capacity to work in a more democratic way.

Kate had initially responded very positively to the move, taking more care over her appearance, going out regularly to visit her parents and to work in the day centre. After several months, she complained of feeling terribly lethargic and staff felt that she appeared depressed. In staff meetings, the problem was discussed and it was agreed that she may be feeling depressed after the initial raising of expectations on leaving hospital. The community psychiatrist visited and advised that her depot medication and 'side-effect' tablets be reduced since the dose was making her too sleepy. Despite this thinking and the cautious approach that had been taken to the move, however, staff were told to threaten her with a return to hospital if she did not 'keep things up'.

Jane, in contrast, was seen as a problem for being too independent in her ideas and activities. Her refusal to attend the day centre was reported and discussed repeatedly. After an argument with another resident over some missing clothes, staff were advised to approach her about the possibility of moving on. Although she had shown interest in a more independent lifestyle, rather than the subject being suggested to her gradually, as a positive step, it was presented as a result of problems in the house and so was perceived by her as being like an ultimatum.

I asked Jane how things were going in the house. She was rather confused about it and not very happy. She felt there was pressure on her to move. The staff had brought up the subject several times and she felt it was unfair, as though everything was being put onto her. She felt this was partly because she was seen as the more independent person.

She did not move, although staff continued to report her attitude to day care as a problem, and she continued to feel under pressure. Some time later, she spoke about this feeling again: Jane told me about what the staff had said — that she was the only one to question things. She said that she had met one man in another group home who seemed frightened to do so. She explained that 'once you've been in an institution you carry it with you, and there is always fear, especially fear that you can be sent back in'. She is aware that the staff may try to use this fear.

Ambivalence about leaving is not only experienced by residents, therefore, but by the staff of the hospital whose demise is presented unambiguously by the departure. Even the group-home staff, who contrasted their role to that of nurses as being rehabilitative and caring rather than custodial, experienced contradictions in their approach towards community care. It seemed that they were attempting to facilitate change and to order it, while being encouraged to regard the patients' situation as essentially unalterable.

LIVING IN A GROUP HOME

Group homes

Among the range of alternative services developed to replace the hospitals, group homes could be said to exemplify the common aims of care in the community. They are always shared housing, varying in levels of support from those with visiting staff to those with 24-hour nursing staff. They can also be closely compared with residential care for other client groups, which, despite a common professional view that services reflect the characteristics of their clients, are markedly similar in basic pattern (e.g. Willcocks *et al.*, 1987). One of the key principles behind group-home development is that of mutual support, practical and social, between residents. In this and many other cases, the principle is taken to the point of seeing the group home as a substitute family.

In the closure process, Health and Local Authorities have been involved in providing group homes and small hostels, but the majority of projects have been developed and managed by voluntary organizations in co-operation with them. On the whole, capital funding for the buildings comes from external sources, such as Housing Association grants, while revenue funding for salaries, running and housekeeping costs comes from resident fees that are set at DSS benefit limits and topped-up by grants from the Health Authority.

The organization providing the group homes studied here had previously run unstaffed group homes in each district, together with a day centre and a network of evening clubs run by volunteers. The existing services had been relatively poorly funded and so would not have been considered for the longer-term patients who would need greater staff support. The organization was well established, therefore, with a strong ethos of charitable work. It was managed by a small and stable managerial group acting for a board of trustees.

The way in which the homes in this study were designed was informed by something akin to normalization principles. The voluntary organization regarded this as commonsense: a straightforward idea of homeliness and ordinariness. This was set in conscious opposition to features of hospital design, which can be seen as 'institutional' and counter to rehabilitation. So, the group homes have a rehabilitation function, but they were not viewed as transitional or a stage in return to more independent living, but as 'homes for life'. We will later examine how coherent this principle is, seen from the residents' perspective.

Everyday life in group homes

The main features of the design, use of space and time and of social interaction in the home can be directly opposed to those found in a long-stay hospital ward. These contrasts were all important in the impression they made on staff and prospective residents. To the staff, they promised a new way of working and residents' progress towards a more ordinary and independent way of life. To prospective residents, it offered a different symbolic valuation of themselves — one that was worth bothering about. I suggest also that these changes had to be understood in a relative sense as there were important continuities with the hospital regime but first let us look at the contrasts which were made and their practical effects.

In the hospital, certain aspects of everyday life, routine, choice, privacy and social relationships, had all been problematic. Long-stay patients had become used to this structure over many years, and professional concerns were focused on whether such institutionalized patients could cope with the loss of imposed structures. Talking to the three groups of patients in my study showed that they could cope with such changes, if given appropriate support. The hospital regime had simply been something to put up with.[5]

For the three projects, four houses were bought and modernized, to provide accommodation for a total of 20 people. Two small houses formed one project, with two groups of four residents living as close neighbours, supported by a single staff group based in one house. The second project was a medium-sized house, for four people, about a mile from the first project. The third was a large Victorian family house, which was large enough to cater for seven residents, all with single bedrooms and with sleeping-in as well as office facilities for staff. They ranged therefore from the most independent home, the small house without an integral office base, to the larger home that was set up with 24-hour staffing and higher ratios to cater for people with higher dependency. This home was, as a result, the least 'family-like' or ordinary in character.

The homes were all modernized to a good Housing Association standard, retaining the original room layout. They used normal domestic fittings, except for the rather intrusive fire safety systems.[6] Private space was provided by residents' bedrooms and communal space in the living room and kitchen. The majority of residents were able to choose a single room, but a few were obliged (or able if they chose) to share. Residents were not allowed to have room keys, however, ostensibly because this was not seen by managers to fit with a family environment. These two features, however well-intended, did not take into account the fact that many residents, even coming from the same hospital wards, felt themselves to be virtual strangers.

---

[5] A demographic study of the population of the two hospitals shows that these groups were typical of long-stay patients (TAPS, 1988). However, they might be distinguished by their willingness to leave hospital, early in the closure process.
[6] Registered care home regulations can in some ways contradict the design of the environment around rehabilitation or normalization principles, since they do not allow for risk-taking as part of development.

The use of space in the homes, therefore, aside from the staff facilities, was much like that of ordinary housing, even though the housing was shared: residents could cook, do their own laundry, care for and use their own rooms, or even tend a plot in the garden. The aim was to create a domestic environment that facilitated everyday activities and residents' sense of pride in their living environment.

Daily routines

The daily routine in group homes did not differ radically from that of the ward, but was generally more flexible, allowing a more adult lifestyle. Residents chose their own rising times and bedtimes, but otherwise the day was structured to some extent by the conventions of the home and of day care. Residents were expected to be up in time to attend a day centre, to limit time spent in their rooms (particularly in bed) and to co-operate with communal evening meal arrangements.

The flexibility of everyday routines was profoundly affected by the nature of daytime activities available and was chosen by staff. Several residents continued to attend the hospital's industrial therapy unit. In two homes, the majority of residents attended a similar local unit. Thus, apart from the movement between home and day centre by public transport, the pattern of their days was still contained within a psychiatric frame. In the third home, in a neighbouring borough, more use was made of informal facilities such as a drop-in club for service users and non-segregated education and leisure facilities, so that the residents' lifestyles appeared more flexible and consequently more 'normal'. Interestingly, this was the larger home, intended for people with a 'higher dependency', yet residents were able to pursue more varied local activities. It is clear from this that activity was not simply constrained by the problems of the residents themselves, but by the limited confidence or vision of those providing care.

Within the home, domestic facilities enabled residents to make more choices in the most basic daily needs, which had become restricted in hospital. They were able to make their own breakfast, in their own time, for example. Although a fairly strict rota operated for housework and cooking communal evening meals, staff aimed to encourage residents to choose what to buy and cook, as well as to help them in doing this. Generally, residents were enabled and encouraged to make everyday choices that fitted reasonably well with the aims of the home. Scope for choices in larger areas of life, such as who to share a room or the home with, was not generally available, unless the resident's preference was seen to follow the lines of organizational preference or need.

Domestic activity was, therefore, a route to giving residents everyday choices as well as towards greater independence. Since staff thinking was so centred on domestic work, it also came to be a key means of structuring the days and weeks, alongside medication and day care, in attempting to order residents' lives. Shared tasks were used by staff as the main basis for social interaction with residents and attempting to supervise interaction among residents.

The work of staff was described as 'groupwork'. This does not indicate a psychological or psychodynamic orientation, but a guiding rule that staff should work with residents and encourage them to 'gell' as a group. Group activities were generally preferred to those initiated and followed individually. Within this the aim was to foster residents' abilities to care for themselves, and for the group, by doing things with rather than for them. So, while in the hospital residents felt staff had done things to them, the intention here was that residents would learn, within limits, to do things with and for others.

I have already touched on the way in which the design of the homes enabled a use of space markedly different to that of the hospital ward. The room layout meant that life did not have to be conducted on a large-group scale, with little individual differentiation. There was a strong emphasis, however, on the desirability of residents using communal facilities. Long hours spent in bedrooms was generally interpreted as a sign of problems within the individual or group. Residents could make their own snacks and drinks, but here the preference of staff for shared activity was reinforced by some residents, who placed a high value on the communal pot of tea, as opposed to the single teabag.

Having personal bedrooms was the key to personal privacy for residents and had been enshrined in policy by one of the two District Health Authorities involved. As a result, one project was allocated the additional funding to ensure that all residents could have their own room, even though the availability of two double rooms made the choice to share possible. In the other homes, two of the residents were obliged to share, but this was handled, fortunately, through the policy of encouraging friends to leave hospital together, if both were deemed suitable by the caring agencies. So, for some residents, shared bedrooms provided a mixture of privacy and company, while the others had their own space for the first time in many years. One resident initially told me that she did not mind a dormitory, she had got used to it, but after about a year in the home told me how much she appreciated her own room. She commented that the smaller scale of the home pushed people together much more and that this could be stressful. She liked to go to her own room to read, or to be alone, as well as to sit in the living room to watch TV or for company.

Homes for life?

On moving, having been told that these were homes for life, residents were encouraged to feel this was their own home. This notion was contradicted, however, by basic conditions of their running and management. Residents were unable to choose their own furniture or room decorations, apparently due to the delays of the selection process. Residents' autonomy and the image of ordinariness was inevitably affected by the presence of a staff office in all but one home. Staff were not constantly present as they had been in hospital since, in all but one home, they worked a 10-hour day and were often out shopping, attending meetings or visiting other homes. The office, unlike a ward's glass-panelled nursing station, did not encourage staff to sit and watch over residents at a distance. Nonetheless, the residents became aware that they were still under continual observation: several commented that staff were always writing notes to report to managers on their behaviour.[7]

When talking to Jane about staff/resident relations in the home, she said that she could appreciate why they had to write reports but did not like the way it was used, like a threat, the feeling of it being like at school: 'it's like it's come full circle — like being told to get up and go out by your parents ...'

On balance, therefore, the group home enhanced the residents' privacy and feelings of dignity, but the degree of privacy afforded was limited by organizational constraints and the continuing position of residents as psychiatric patients.

Relationships between residents were also crucial, since the home environment enabled them to support each other but to some extent threw them together in this way. Residents did a great deal for and with each other and more able residents were relied upon to help others out. Brian, for example, often made breakfast for all the residents before staff came on duty; Mary did a larger share of the shopping for her house and cooked extras such as home-baked cakes for residents and visitors; Joan did the main share of the housework in her home because, she said, she needed to busy herself in the house and could not stand the messiness of some residents. As in any normal domestic situation, the sharing of chores and space led to both mutual help and tensions between residents. Although staff tended to focus on such tensions as problems, they could be interpreted positively, as reflecting a higher and more 'normal' level of social interaction.

Living in a hospital ward led to a curious mixture of living in communal space, under continual observation — a sort of public life — and a lack of communal integration. Generally, in hospitals the level of social activity is low, and social interaction among patients often takes place away from the ward, in neutral spaces. The residents of one group home described to me how they had hardly known each other before the preparations to move out of hospital together began, despite years of living on the same ward. Similarly, they did not feel close to nursing staff, although certain

---

[7] Their response to the research was acceptance and in some cases strong support. I hoped that they would see my role as reporting their views rather than reporting on them in the manner of case notes.

individuals — the ones who were adaptable and attentive who might sit and chat to you — were remembered as 'good nurses'.

Friendships based in the hospital had been few and fragile — Hilda and Mary kept up links with two fellow patients who had also left hospital, but none of the residents returned to the ward to visit old friends. The residents were a fairly elderly group of people, reflecting an average length of hospital stay of 21+ years. They had been and remained fairly isolated, even though they were not the most socially isolated among the hospital population. Of the 20 residents, eight had lost all contact with family or friends out of hospital. After a year of living in the group homes, this situation had not changed. Six of the residents had some remaining contacts, which were generally very occasional or fragile. The other six residents had managed to maintain regular contact with one or more relatives and the majority were able to return to their former local area where some relatives still lived.

Moving to a group home had the greatest social impact on the second group, by providing a home ground that appeared more normal and was more amenable to sociability. Doris, for example, felt that her relatives had stopped coming to see her because of the stigma of where she was. It was too late, after all these years, for radical changes, but she did begin to exchange letters with her sister. Jane went to visit the brother she had not seen for years, and her son and grandchildren became regular visitors to the house. Apart from relatives, none of the residents had social contacts outside the psychiatric sphere, and living in a group home did little to alter this pattern. The residents themselves lacked the confidence to go out and look for friends and they were not encouraged to do so except within the network of homes and day centres created by the voluntary organization.

Staff attitudes to families were also ambiguous. Although they welcomed occasional visits, for tea and for special occasions, very frequent visits into or out of the home were responded to as an imposition. I will explore what may lie behind such staff practices when describing the family model of care.

Continuities with hospital life

It is clear, therefore, that despite the reforms that were given careful attention in design and approach, residents experienced significant continuities with their status as hospital patients. My argument is that resistance to change was reinforced by several basic features of the organization and philosophy of care through which the alternative facilities were shaped. I will outline some important aspects of group home life that were relatively similar to those of hospital life and then go on to examine some of the factors that have contributed to the reproduction of organizational cultures in this way.

Medication

The use of medication in the home indicates an important continuity with hospital life. Firstly, it places paramedical and supervisory responsibilities on staff who otherwise see their role as one of social care. New staff members sometimes reacted against medication policy, but the in-house training and the patterns of communication between older and newer staff on the job encouraged them to gradually internalize policies on this and other matters as being necessary and right. Just as in hospital, the medication round was integral to the structuring of time and activity, in the home staff aimed to establish a regular routine.

All the residents were on some form of psycho-active medication; the majority receiving major tranquillizers by tablets or depot injections, plus 'anti side-effect tablets'. Those patients who had received some training on self-administered medication, in preparation for leaving, returned to a system controlled by staff. Similarly, although residents were allocated GPs after leaving, who were responsible for prescribing, managers generally frowned on any attempt to alter the pattern established in hospital.

The understanding imparted to staff was that medication was what made community care possible, so that regular medication was essential to order and control in the home. In this way, it took on a treatment function and was not simply an ordinary house. Although some workers were uncomfortable with this role, and on a 10-hour shift were practically unable to monitor all medication closely, they were taught to associate stability with medication and relapse of psychiatric symptoms with lack of medication. Knowledge of common side-effects was vague and staff generally interpreted resident complaints about these as due to unco-operativeness or lack of insight into their condition and the benefits of medication. Residents continued to receive minimal information on their medications and were not given any trust or responsibility in this area.

Day care

The reliance on day care as part of group-home management was particularly problematic from the residents' perspective. Although types of psychiatric day centre vary from informal clubs to highly structured centres with a therapeutic or work base, three of the homes were in a borough where existing facilities were limited. Since the hospital closure process had not yet dealt with the issue of daytime activities, all these residents were expected to return to the hospital industrial therapy unit or to use a similar day centre run by the voluntary organization. During a series of day visits to the centre, I participated in the packaging work, with residents, and heard their views of the centre. The work was fiddly but relatively simple and very repetitive. Much of the possibility for enjoyment would come from talking to other members, and several people commented that it was this that made the work worthwhile. Others, however, commented on the very low level of social interaction that I had observed.

From a professional and organizational viewpoint there was a clear set of reasons for insisting that all residents should attend a centre. Day care was viewed as an alternative to employment, which was not considered possible for these individuals. As such it would offer some of the benefits of occupation: prevention of boredom, a work ethic and feelings of self worth.[8] It was also a means of separating spheres of activity such as home and work. Although going to the day centre could function, like a job, as something to 'get you out of the house', the separation was within the psychiatric system. Residents used public transport, not to get to ordinary local facilities such as community centres, but to segregated ones.

Although the work done was paid, the rate was nominal. The majority felt it offered them merely pocket money and they derived little pride or independence from this. The work itself was felt by all members I spoke with to be boring and inherently unrewarding, but they would often point out that it was better than nothing. One or two residents took some pride, however, in doing something useful. The rationale for such day care conflicted with the fact that the majority of residents were of retirement age. Several residents pointed this out clearly and logically to staff, adding that they found the centre boring and did not see why they should not be entitled to retirement like any normal person. Group-home staff agreed with this view, but found that managers would not support it, unless alternative structured day care could be obtained. This reflects two other rationales: firstly, the belief that psychiatric patients, if allowed to be inactive, will relapse into symptoms such as hearing voices; secondly, the need of the organization is to have residents provided with structured activity during the day.

Ironically, when considering the homes' emphasis on rehabilitation, those residents who wished to pursue more independent activities were repeatedly reported as problems. An unwillingness to fit with the official ideal was regarded as evidence of problems within the person, rather than problems in relating to a limited regime. Mary, for example, was very active within the home, and enjoyed going out when she was in a positive mood. She found the day centre unsuitable and unenjoyable. One member of staff suggested she might be happier with the local pensioners' lunch club, but this was never followed up. The problem was regarded as hers, a reflection of her personality. This worker eventually persuaded the Local Authority to offer her, and another elderly resident, a part-time place in a day centre for elderly people which focused more on social and leisure activities. This she found more congenial, even though, as she said, 'they treat you like an invalid'.

---

[8] This rationale is striking in its similarity to the ideas of the 19th century moral management approach, related by Skultans, 1979.

Jane's main interest was in painting and writing. She did not want to work, especially in such an unrewarding role, and told me that she had been branded 'difficult and unco-operative' in hospital, for her refusal to attend industrial therapy. She expressed interest in attending art classes at a local community centre but lacked the confidence to start going alone. When this was raised in a staff meeting the manager said he was doubtful about residents attending non-psychiatric facilities.

In order to understand the reasons for these sort of conflicts, between the aim of rehabilitation and a more ordinary life, and the management of issues such as medication, residents' activities and major choices, we have to look at the structures and attitudes that shaped everyday practice. The following paragraphs explore some of the factors in the resistance to change and democracy that the residents experienced.

Voluntary organizations generally differ from statutory bodies in terms of scale and organizational style. Many have grown from small, localized groups, often focused around a particular interest or need and became involved in service provision through perceiving a gap in public services or the need for a new approach. Voluntary organizations providing mental health care tend to operate on a limited scale and provide smaller-scale facilities than statutory agencies. They regard their position as closer to the community, either a local area or a community of interest, than that of large institutions such as hospitals, and also as being more directly responsive to users' needs.

However, recent policy developments, such as hospital closure plans and the development of contracting plans following the NHS and Community Care Act 1990, have drawn voluntary organizations into mainstream service provision. The impact on the organizations managing these group homes is instructive. The management had traditionally been by a small and stable group. Care staff have no formal means of contributing to decision-making, but in the past, with very small numbers of staff and larger numbers of volunteers, this had taken place in an informal way. The numbers of paid care staff rose dramatically in a two-year period, due to the reprovision projects, so that administrative, management and training demands on the organization grew rapidly.

Its structure was not unlike that of the hospitals, but with a shallower and less elaborate hierarchy. Care staff (like hospital nurses) felt they had little say in policy or practice decisions, despite their greater personal knowledge of residents. The feelings staff expressed to me personally, and in shared discussions, indicated that this was a source of dissatisfaction. Alongside this, a perceived lack of attention to their training and development led to some frustration. The main recruitment policy was to select people on the basis of a caring and stable personality, with an interest in the work, rather than requiring qualifications or experience. Managers saw this as a positive policy, since care was perceived as natural and intuitive, something that could be spoilt by professionalization.

Models of group-home life

The gendered hierarchy of the hospital extends into group-home management and lifestyle through the use of a family model as a guiding philosophy. The model is one of a substitute family where carers are viewed in a quasi-maternal role, their managers as paternal and the residents as childlike. This imagery bears a direct relation to the ways in which patients were selected for community living, with a focus on dependency categories, and to the way in which group homes are designed and managed.

The family principle fits neatly with the use of domesticity and an ordinary home environment in rehabilitation, even though we have seen that in important ways the environment was not ordinary. It also fits comfortably with the rather vague notions of community and of caring that have been outlined. The 'as-if' family can be seen as an alternative basis for community, which avoids the need for staff to support residents in approaching the difficult issue of integration in the wider community. We have seen that social interaction was encouraged primarily through sharing in the home and through contacts within the quasi-kinship network of group homes and day centres. The notion of community offered is based on kinship, but an exclusively psychiatric one, with boundaries drawn by categories of deviancy.

Motherhood can be viewed, in opposition to the custodianship that the hospitals have been seen to represent, as a benign form of caring and controlling. It can also mask the real inequalities that are characteristic of family and of wider social groupings. In a sense, the family was also a model for relationships between social groups with differential power. The residents were not only seen as childlike but as stereotypically lower class — industrial therapy was seen as appropriate to their social standing, for example, in a way which painting or going to the theatre was not.

The model also ignores the fact that the residents have had, and often continue to have, families of their own. Such relationships were significant to them, even where they were now damaged or broken by hospitalization and the crises that preceded it. In accounts of their past lives, residents spoke mainly about their families, with a vividness and recollection that contrasted starkly with their recollections of events and people in hospital. It was as though the entry to hospital was a sort of ending and the period of life in hospital a timeless limbo (Hazan, 1980). A few residents had spent all their adult lives in institutions — like Jean who was admitted to the hospital at the age of 16 years and never left, and Joe, who had been admitted after spending his first adult years in the Army. The majority of the female residents, however, unlike the men, had married and had children before being admitted to hospital.

The passage below from one resident's account of her history gives some insight:

'... *The GP told me I must get a job if I was to get over the depression and I found one in a school canteen. But then dad got worse, falling over. The doctor said he couldn't put him in hospital; then a few days later a woman doctor came and agreed to admit him so that I could keep my job. He died the next week. I felt guilty because he'd cursed me for putting him in hospital, even though I felt it was the only thing to do. I know he would have died anyway. He was 95 and very ill. I suppose my life was ended at that time, in a way.'*

The notion of the patient as childlike is not unique to group homes, or indeed to psychiatry. Hockey and James (1988), for example, describe how elderly people in residential care are overwhelmingly viewed by carers as like children and infantilized by them. (See also Alasewski (1986) on mental handicap services.) These attitudes are more widely linked to the dependency status of people who are receiving personal care, but are also found in the ideas of care staff about the nature of mental illness. The ideas of community and hospital-based workers are complex, relying on much more than a biomedical theory (Perelberg, 1985), and the dominant view imparted to group-home workers was of people who have become stuck at or regressed to an immature stage of development.

Residents' perception

It is important to be aware that the group home, a family home, was not conceived to be the residents' own. Not only was selection for a particular home dependent on professional judgements, and relatively passive resident acceptance or choice, but residents were not afforded any tenancy rights. So, although the group home is described as a 'home for life', security depends on the psychiatric categorization of the person. It depends on professional discretion rather than rights.

The three female residents of one home confronted this issue when staff, after a year in the home, became involved in selection of two further residents. Although staff and residents were told that their views would be taken into account, residents' attempts to argue that they did not want any male residents were regarded as silly. Managers attempted to explain their views away as a result of psychiatric problems and an inability to accept change of any type. Care staff were instructed to persuade the residents to accept the two men who were being considered and, after several months of arguing their viewpoint, they realized that they had no say in the matter. The decision was taken regardless of their feelings or even of care staff attempts to support their views. This case revealed to the residents in what ways the home was not their own. It provides a reflection on the basic contradictions in trying to create a reformed system of community care, without altering the basic attitudes that define the residents' moral and social status.

Problem definition and resolution

We have looked, at various points, at the ways in which particular individuals were defined as problematic and at particular issues around which problems tended to be defined. The pattern of recognizing and resolving such problems suggests that definition from a management perspective tends to mask the patterns of conflict between staff and residents and also between home-based staff/residents and centrally-based managers.

The language with which problems were reported and discussed in staff meetings shows how clinical categories such as 'mania' (which are themselves derived from wider cultural concepts) were used situationally and interchangeably with lay categories such as 'low'. Whether a person in difficulties is treated as ill, childish, unhappy or simply experiencing ordinary problems is influenced by the role of that person within the home and the acceptability or deviancy of his/her behaviour within the norms of its regime. So, care staff and managers may 'play down' distress experienced by residents, or fall back on a punitive use of diagnostic labels and assumptions when a resident's behaviour seems to threaten the established order of the group home. In this way, staff have the authority to redefine the resident's viewpoint. A shared complaint, for example, can be dismissed by individualizing the problem — 'you're the only one to question things' — yet categorizing the person — she's a manic, she can't cope with making decisions'.

As recipients of psychiatric services, these individuals were in a situation where they seemed inherently unable to do the right thing. While people in a sick role are expected to co-operate with healers and return to a normal social role, psychiatric patients find themselves unable, by definition, to do so, since the state of mental illness itself is defined in terms of an apparent deviation from normal social roles. Similarly, the residents found they were exhorted to co-operate with rehabilitation, in order to progress towards a more independent and ordinary life, in a system in which ordinary expectations and actions could result in being redefined as sick.

While the services had shifted to a community location and a reforming philosophy that was guided by ideas of kinship and caring, the residents found themselves essentially marooned within the community.

RE-EVALUATING THE PAST

The case history

Before concluding and in order to understand further the dilemmas faced by care staff in this setting, I want to return to the ways in which residents were selected to move to the group homes. In a sense, we can draw a thread from the history of the asylums and the policy of community care, through the hospital closure plans to the current predicaments of individual former patients. The forms of knowledge that professionals relied upon were problematical. Clinical history is an illness history and one that is not oriented towards the (supposed) current aims of rehabilitation change and restoration. As such, the clinical history is even a partial illness history, since it arises out of the reduction and reification of the person that has taken place.

In order to address this imbalance, which appears like an great empty space in the lives of these people once the closure is faced, we need to look more to personal and social history and to the way in which the residents themselves recall and restructure their lives.

The life history

The accounts by residents of their own lives revealed the complexity and vividness that had been missing from their official histories. These were, on the whole, ordinary lives, but which had been marked by extraordinary losses. As Mary once said, 'I'm grieving, but for something else'. Their life histories reflect a preoccupation with the process of change (one that was absent from staff approaches to leaving hospital) returning to a more integrated past, of childhood and earlier family or working life, and exploring the events that led to the present.

Unlike the case history, these show the residents as being involved in differing roles over their lifetimes and having insight into their own experiences. The theme of women's experience of life is strong, as is the significance of the experience of war, leading to grief, separation and fear. They show ways in which the residents tried to make sense of their lives. There is an impression that, because so much of their lives has been taken away — the loss of home, of family and ordinary identity — they needed to talk about other periods of life that were important to them. The ordinary side of the self as well as the losses and problems are revealed.

In these histories (in direct opposition to the case histories) the hospital phase of life is reduced, appearing almost empty in some ways. It is not the case that the residents tried to ignore or to forget their lives in the institution, but a reflection of its lack of value for them, its very emptiness in the course of their lives. The transition from hospital to group home is not, however, a reversal of the process involved in becoming a patient. The moral and social position of the patients was not transformed in the way it had been on entry to hospital, despite all the benefits of the move that they experienced.

If the aim of the closure was to achieve a re-integration of 'chronic' psychiatric patients into their own community, rehabilitation needed to be more than a matter of training in living skills and to become a rounded and self-sustaining process. In order for the residents to redevelop a positive self-image, carers must be able to form such an image themselves, of the patients as people.

SUMMARY AND CONCLUDING POINTS

So, we cannot assume that transition is simple, a matter of changing places, when this ignores the history of the institution and of the patient's experience. If de-institutionalization is the aim of hospital closure, then we need to consider the way patients view themselves and how their experience relates to the continuing or changing power relations in the institution and in the world outside.

From this critical analysis it may seem easy to form a negative view of the hospital-closure process, but it should be clear that transition led (as it should have done) to raised expectations among many patients. The research has shown something of the great improvements that were achieved, in the objective and subjective quality of life of those leaving. These are achievements that can be built upon by staff and residents working together. The majority of this group of residents, after 2.5 years, were still living in the group homes, with the mixture of contentment and dispute that any ordinary life affords. One resident has moved on to a sheltered council flat and one resident returned to hospital during the initial trial period, opting to try a move to a different home. Except for two residents, who had mixed feelings about the move, all were glad to have left hospital and did not want to return.

This section raises, however, several issues to be tackled in policy and practice. It argues particularly that democratization, and a related change in the status of giving and receiving care, needs to be pursued throughout all levels of service provision. Many working examples exist of how this can be done. Several establishments now give residents basic tenancy rights, involve both care staff and residents in developmental training and give them voices in decision-making. (For further ideas of alternative models for residential care see Brandon (1981) and Barker and Peck (1988).)

This account shows not only what some of the continuing issues may be in the transition to community-based care, but also something of what can be achieved by the residents and those who work with and care for them.

SUGGESTIONS FOR FURTHER READING

Brandon, D. (1981) *Voices of Experience: Consumer Perspectives of Psychiatric Treatment*. London, MIND.

Goldie, N. (1988) *"I hated it there but I miss the people. A study of what has happened to a group of ex long-stay patients from Claybury hospital.'* South Bank Polytechnic, Health and Social Services Research Unit. In a series of interviews, former residents of Claybury hospital talk about their experiences of leaving and living outside.

Islington Mental Health Forum (1989) *Fit for Consumption? Mental Health Users' Views of Treatment in Islington*. IMHF, London. (Available from MIND mail order service, London.)

Thomas, D. and Rose N. *Getting to Know You*. A reflection and review of an individualized approach to service planning, Manchester Health Authority, 1986 — an example and guide to using the approach first set out by Brost and Johnson.

'What Matters Most' is a training pack centred on putting yourself in the service user's shoes, devised by Kent University in collaboration with South East

London Regional Health Authority. Packs are currently available for work with elderly people and people with learning difficulties, but would be appropriate for wider use.

Wolfensberger, W. and Glenn, T. (1975) *PASS: Programme Analysis of Service Systems.* National Institute for Mental Retardation, Toronto. *'PASS'* was originally devised for service evaluation. Several models are now available for use by service providers and training courses based on PASS are advertised from time to time in OPENMIND magazine.

REFERENCES

Abrahamson, D. and Bremer, D. (1982) Do long-stay patients want to leave hospital? *Health Trends*, **14**, 95–7.

Abrams, P., Abrams S., Humphrey, R. and Snaith R. (1986) *Neighbourhood Care and Social Policy.* HMSO, London.

Alasewski, A. (1986) *Institutional Care and the Mentally Handicapped.* Croom Helm, London.

Banton, R., Clifford, P., Frosch, S., Lousada, J. and Rosenthall, J. (1985) *The Politics of Mental Health.* Macmillan, London.

Barker, I. and Peck, E. (1988) (eds.) *Power in Strange Places.*, Good Practices in Mental Health, London.

Barton, R. (1959) *Institutional Neurosis*, Wright, Bristol,

Baruch, G. and Treacher, A. (1978) *Psychiatry Observed.* Routledge, London.

Basaglia, F. (1982) Breaking the circuit of control. In: Ingleby, D. (ed.) *Critical Psychiatry*. Penguin, Harmondsworth.

Booth, T., Simons, K. and Booth, W. (1990) *Outward Bound: Relocation and Community Care for People with Learning Difficulties.* Open University Press, Milton Keynes.

Bourdieu, P. (1972) *Outline of a Theory of Practice.* Cambridge University Press, Cambridge.

Brost, M. and Johnson, T. (1982) *Getting to Know You.* Wisconsin Coalition for Advocacy and New Concepts for the Handicapped Inc., Madison, Wisconsin.

Brown, G.W. and Harris, T. (1978) *Social Origins of Depression: A Study of Psychiatric Disorder in Women.* Tavistock, London.

Bulmer, M. (1986) *Neighbours: The Work of Philip Abrams.* Cambridge University Press, Cambridge.

Bulmer, M. (1987) *The Social Basis of Community Care.* Allen and Unwin, London.

Busfield, J. (1986) *Managing Madness: Changing Ideas and Practice.* Hutchison, London.

Carson, J. (1988) *The Hall and Baker Rehabilitation Survey of Claybury Hospital.* TAPS, Unpublished data.

Cohen, A. (1989) *Creating community: An Anthropological Study of Psychiatric Care in Bologna*, Italy 1960–87, PhD London School of Economics.

DHSS and CPA (1987) *Home Life: A Code of Practice for Residential Care.* A report of a working party sponsored by the DHSS and convened by CPA under the chairmanship of Kina, Lady Avebury. Centre for Policy on Ageing, London.

DOH (1989) *Caring for People. Community Care in the Next Decade and Beyond.* HMSO, London, Cmnd. 849.

Dingwall, R. (1976) *Aspects of Illness.* Martin Robertson, London.

Douglas, M. (1974) *Purity and Danger: An Analysis of Concepts of Pollution and Taboo.* Routledge and Kegan Paul, London.

Douglas, M. (1987) *How Institutions Think.* Routledge, London.

Evans-Pritchard, E. (1937) *Oracles, Witchcraft and Magic among the Azande.* Cambridge University Press, Cambridge.

Finch, J. and Groves, D. (1983) *A Labour of Love: Women, Work and Caring.* Routledge, London.

Foucault, M. (1967) *Madness and Civilisation: A History of Insanity in the Age of Reason.* Tavistock, London.

Foucault, M. (1979) *Discipline and Punish: the Birth of the Prison.* Penguin, Harmondsworth.

Garfinkel, H. (1956) Conditions of successful degradation ceremonies, *American Journal of Sociology*, **61**, 72–95.

Geertz, C. (1973) *The Interpretation of Cultures: Selected Essays*, Basic Books, New York.

Goffman, E. (1967) *Where the Action Is.* Penguin, Harmondsworth.

Goffman, E. (1968) *Asylums: Essays on the Social Situation of Mental Patients and Other Inmates.* Penguin, Harmondsworth.

Goffman, E. (1971) *The Presentation of Self in Everyday Life.* Penguin, Harmondsworth.

Griffiths, Sir Roy (1988) *Community Care: An Agenda for Action — A Report to the Secretary of State for Social Services.* HMSO, London.

Hazan, H. (1980) *The Limbo People. A Study of the Constitution of the Time Universe Among the Aged.* Routledge, London.

Hockey, J. and James, A. (1988) *Growing up and growing old: Metaphors of ageing in contemporary Britain*, ASA Conference Papers.

Ingleby, D. (ed.) (1981) *Critical Psychiatry: The Politics of Mental Health.* Penguin, Harmondsworth.

Jones, K. (1972) *The History of the Mental Health Services.* Routledge and Kegan Paul, London.

King's Fund (1980) *An Ordinary Life. Project Paper No. 24.* King's Fund, London.

Kleinman, A. (1980) *Patients and Healers in the Context of Culture: An Exploration of the Borderland between Anthropology, Medicine and Psychiatry.* University of California Press, Berkeley.

Korman, N. and Glennerster, H. (1985) *Closing a Hospital: The Darenth Park Project.* Bedford Square Press, London.

Korman, N. and Glennerster, H. (1990) *Hospital Closure: A Political and Economic Study.* Open University Press, Milton Keynes.

Kuhn, T.S. (1970) *The Structure of Scientific Revolutions*, 2nd edn. University of Chicago Press, Chicago.

Lewin, E. and Olesen, V. (eds.) (1985) *Women, Health and Healing.* Tavistock, London.

Mangen, S. and Rao, B. (eds.) (1985) *Mental Health Care in the European Community.* Croom Helm, London.

Marris, P. (1974) *Loss and Change.* Routledge, London.

McLaughlin, M. (1990) *The Friern Report: An Experiment in Resettlement.* Peter Bedford Trust, London.

Menzies-Lyth, I. (1970) *The Functioning of Social Systems as a Defence Against Anxiety.* Tavistock, London.

Murray Parkes, C. (1971) Psychosocial transitions: A field for study. *Social Science and Medicine*, **5**, 101–15.

NETRHA (1982) *The Future Provision of Services for the Mentally Ill: A Consultative Document.* NETRHA, London.

Parsons, T. (1951) *The Social System.* Free Press, New York.

Perelberg, R. J. (1985) *Family and Mental Illness in a London Borough.* PhD. London School of Economics.

Perrucci, R. (1974) *Circle of Madness: On Being Insane and Institutionalized in America.* Prentice-Hall, New Jersey.

Ramon, S. (1985) *Psychiatry in Britain: Meaning and Policy*. Croom Helm, London.
Ramon, S. (1990) Symbolic interaction perspectives on leaving hospital. *Social Work and Social Science Review*, **1**(3), 163–176.
Ramon, S. and Giannichedda, M. G. (1988) *Psychiatry in Transition: British and Italian Experiences*. Pluto Press, London
Rosenhan, D. (1973) On being sane in insane places. *Science*, **179**, 250–8.
Scull, A. (1977) *Decarceration: Community Treatment and the Deviant: A Radical View*. Prentice-Hall, Englewood Cliffs.
Sinclair, I. (ed.) (1988) *Residential Care, The Research Reviewed*. Literature surveys commissioned by the independent review of residential care, chaired by Gillian Wagner. HMSO, London.
Skultans, V. (1979) *English Madness. Ideas on Insanity 1580–1890*. Routledge, London.
Stacey M. (1988) *The Sociology of Health and Healing*. Unwin Hyman, London.
TAPS (1988) *Preliminary Report on Baseline Data from Friern and Claybury Hospitals*. TAPS, London.
Taussig, M. T. (1980) Reification and the consciousness of the patient. *Social Science and Medicine*, **14B**, 3–13.
Van Gennep A. (1960) *The Rites of Passage*. Routledge, London
Wagner, Lady G. (1988) *A Positive Choice: Report of the Independent Review of Residential Care*. HMSO, London.
Walker, A. (ed.) (1982) *Community Care: The Family, the State and Social Policy*. Blackwell, Oxford.
Willcocks, D., Peace, S. and Kellaher, L. (1987) *Private Lives in Public Places. A Research-based Critique of Residential Life in Local Authority Old People's Homes*. Tavistock, London.
Willmot, P. (1986) *Social Networks, Informal Care and Public Policy*. Policy Studies Institute, London.
Wing, J. and Brown, G. W. (1970) *Institutionalism and Schizophrenia: A Comprehensive Study of Three Mental Hospitals, 1960–68*. Cambridge University Press, Cambridge.
Wolfensberger, W. (1972) *The Principle of Normalization in Human Services*. National Institute of Mental Retardation, Toronto.

Conclusions

Dylan Tomlinson, in Chapter 2, concluded his description of the closure of two psychiatric hospitals by stating that, 'For the moment, this process has left all the major issues for mental health services in the 21st century untouched'. We need to ask ourselves if indeed this is the case, by looking at the major new issues that the closure process has unearthed.

Closure and mental health work as a participative process

The closure of psychiatric hospitals has been described in this book from the perspectives of three of the main contributors to the process: the planners, the professionals, and the service users.

The text highlights that more often than not, these perspectives were in conflict, but that it is possible to find and follow more participative ways of going about the closure. Moreover, to ensure the success of the whole enterprise, it is imperative to search for and select the more participative forms. Conversely, lack of participation and involvement by the main actors in this drama leads to failure to achieve the stated major objectives of hospital closures. However, the reasons for the low level, if not the apparent lack of participation, would need to be more fully understood and tackled if effective participation is to be achieved.

Self-evidently the wish to retain power and the fear of losing it by sharing is at the core of this issue. Secondly, the training of planners and mental health professionals accentuates the view that **each** of them knows best, and that they **should know best**, as a reflection of the widespread belief in the value of expertise. Such beliefs go against the grain of a participative model, which underlies the valid contribution of all of the participants. If anything, the ascendancy of the administrative culture in the 1980s has led to planners being treated, and perceiving themselves, as a dominant **professional** group, assuming unique knowledge and skills, with its own gate-keeping roots (such as the various management courses that each new manager is expected to take after work hours).

Thirdly, so long as the disease model of mental illness continues to be dominant, it will not matter **where** people are treated and whether their perspective is taken on board. Hence de-hospitalization does not necessarily lead to de-institutionalization. A strong belief in the importance of revaluing people who have experienced serious mental distress and in their right to an ordinary life becomes therefore a necessary, but insufficient, condition for the prevention of the re-creation of mini-institutions in the community, and with them an institutionalized way of life.

Fourthly, the various fears of the effects of the closure, raised throughout the book, require serious attention. However, the many examples provided in all of the chapters of reducing these fears do not seem to have led to greater participation among the more dominant British stake holders.

A radical shift of views

In a nutshell, a truly participative model for hospital closure, and for all mental health services, calls for a major and radical shift in our views on the relationships between service providers, service users, and among the different groups of providers. As service users obtain the right to service by being **citizens**, a radical shift in the dominant views on citizenship in each of our societies is required. While recognizing that this would need to be a momentous shift, the current interest in presenting a **citizens' charter** in most First- and Second-world countries, expressed by politicians of most ideological strands, highlights that the relationships between citizens and the state are an issue of concern far beyond the mental health system. The renewed conceptual exploration of citizenship in sociology and social policy reflects a similar trend in which issues of the relationships between the individual and the community, ethnic majority and minority, men and women, are reconsidered within the framework of the state and citizens' rights (Turner, 1990; Yuval-Davis, 1991).

The growing interest in exploring and employing different models of advocacy, including citizen's advocacy and self-advocacy, in some mental health services illustrates another impact of the focus on citizenship (Brandon, 1991, Ch. 6). However, for such a change to be effective at the level of the mental health system, a shift towards a **consumer-led** service and towards **professionals as enablers** rather than as 'the experts', would be necessary. Such a shift is described in several examples outlined in Chapters One, Three and Four. The research methodology used by Christine Perring to follow up the process of resettlement, and the 'inward-looking' approach in the methodology of the research on the social work teams facing the closure of their hospital, provide two more illustrations of how to carry out research that is both consumer-led and attempt to enable the research subjects to express their views and to affect the research findings.

An interesting extension of this direction is reflected in the project on evaluating home care (Youll and Perring, 1991), where the focus is on developing methods that enable users to be frank evaluators of the residential service provided to them (Table 3.3 in Chapter Three).

To experiment with the impact involving users, choose one method of involving users from that table which appeals to you and your co-workers, and which could be feasible within your setting. Try it out at least twice, with an interval of at least two weeks, asking both users

and workers to participate. Set aside time to reflect, for both workers and users, on what you have learned from the experience of using it, as well as from the findings.

The focus on the evaluation of services fits well with the concern for improvement in quality, and in quality control measures. This focus also encourages workers to be more aware of the impact of their methods of work and to have feasible tools for the evaluation of their own contribution. By giving both workers and users such tools 'research' may be demystified and at the same time become accessible as an important tool for taking stock and influencing change in everyday practice. This is not to suggest that there is no place for outsiders as researchers. The 'outsider's' contribution to the 'insiders' brings a different perspective into the equation by virtue of being marginal to the organization.

De-professionalization or re-professionalization?

This issue resurfaces at several junctions such as: (a) the role of non-qualified care staff; (b) the role and identity of professionals in hospital vs. those working in the community; (c) the role and identity during the transitional process; and (d) in leading to a consumer-led service.

Carrier (1990) has suggested that the challenge to professional practice in medicine comes from two directions: (a) from Conservative governments interested in dismantling monopolies on the one hand; and (b) from the 'considerable disillusionment' (p. 121) with professional performance by the informed general public on the other. The fear of the 'disabling professions' expressed since the 1960s has been referred to in Chapter Three.

When applied to mental health, some view a potential move from the traditional role of the professional to that of the enabler as de-professionalization, namely a role in which the professional is discouraged from using his/her knowledge and skills (Jones and Poletti, 1985). Others see this move as re-professionalization, or as an opportunity to focus knowledge and skills on those specific dimensions that cannot be taken care off as well by either service users, informal carers, or paid unqualified carers (Hennelly, 1991; Ramon, 1989). In mental health issues this would include some forms of advice, advocacy, counselling, reaching-out work, networking and supporting people in an acute crisis. In particular, it would imply supporting users, informal carers and unqualified care staff in performing effectively, instead of doing their jobs, yet retaining the flexibility to be able to perform a variety of tasks according to arising needs. Many Italian and British nurses have welcomed the move to work in the community as one of moving from a custodial role to a caring role (De Nicola *et al.*, 1991; Savio, 1991), even though the work in the community has proven to be more demanding.

It is clear that, in a transitional period such as the one in which we are now, cherished past ideas concerning professionalism are doubted and require thorough re-examination as a starting point for effective change. It is equally clear that to be part of such a process is painful, especially if one is left just at the receiving end and is not made an active, involved, partner to the process. This experience parallels the users' experience of being made into passive recipients of the mental health system.

The risk of taking risks

The closure of psychiatric hospitals inevitably leaves an 'empty space' — physically, structurally, socially, conceptually and emotionally. Some of us look forward to empty spaces as offering opportunities for improvement on past traditions and for creativity in doing so. Chapters One, Three, and Four, in particular, offer examples of welcoming such a space. Examples of the fear of such a space and the fear of what change may bring with it also appear in each chapter — especially Chapter Two.

A changing system in which the traditional mode of doing things is questioned calls also for taking calculated risks, recognizing new risks due to change and devising ways of handling them. At the same time it is likely to lead to fear of any risk-taking by some — especially by those standing to lose power due to change. The more significant of these developments are looked at below.

The function of old and new structures

Psychiatric wards in general hospitals and alternative asylums in the community

Psychiatric wards have been portrayed as the new, concrete, site, to replace psychiatric hospitals since their establishment in the 1920s. Most closure plans in the Anglo-Saxon world include an increase in the number of psychiatric beds in the general hospital. They epitomize the treatment of mental distress as another physical illness.

To the observer, most of these are sad places, which lack the bustle of wards for people with physical illness, as the level of technology is much lower and the number of visitors minimal. Only rarely are the wards used to create an atmosphere and a programme that enable people to find better solutions to their problems. Although people come out of these wards after a much shorter time than in a psychiatric hospital, this often happens without sorting out the difficulties for which they were admitted. Symptoms have subsided, but the level of medication has been increased and leavers are often unable to engage in ordinary activities.

Service users, and some professionals, have been advocating that alternative asylum places in the community be established. These are to be low-key, safe houses or 'sanctuaries' in which people will be supported psychologically and physically, rather than medically. People will be able to use these places at a pre-crisis stage, rather than wait for a full-blown crisis to occur (Echlin and Ramon, 1992). The experience of Trieste, in which people can stay in their local community mental health centre and where they interact during the day with other service users beside the staff, provides another possibility of maintaining people in the community even during a crisis, while allowing them and their families to have a 'breathing space' (Dell'Acqua and Mezzina, 1991).

The work of the Naropa Institute in conjunction with the Community Mental Health Centre in Boulder, Colorado, offers another alternative of a safe and supported asylum in the community (Warner, 1991). Cedar House is another facility available in Boulder for people in a mental distress crisis, including psychotic episodes. Here people live in an ordinary middle-class house, with a high ratio of staff per person and a lot of individual attention, leading to a much reduced rate in the use of hospital beds (Warner, 1991). Corby Mental Health Resource Centre offers another response to such a crisis, by being a day facility with an intensive staff input (personal communication), whereas the Barnet intensive crisis intervention interdisciplinary team has demonstrated since 1974 the ability to reduce considerably all hospital admissions, in particular first admissions (Mitchell, 1990).

When the issue of alternative asylums in the community is raised, often the response is 'but what about those dangerous to others and to themselves?' Before we look at this group it is important to remember that it is a small minority, and that its size will become even smaller if such alternatives would exist for the majority which is neither dangerous to itself or to others.

However, this is not an attempt to duck the issue of people who may need a more secure place. For those who offended, a prison with good psychiatric facilities offered by the local community mental health centre may be at times a suitable solution. Being in prison for an offence one admits to have committed, for a fixed term, is about enabling people to continue to be responsible for their actions, even though their mental state is taken into consideration and suitable intervention is provided. For yet others, there may be a need for very small secure units for short periods, as seclusion of any type breeds further frustration and aggression.

Community mental health centres

In the American and Italian visions of a de-hospitalized, de-institutionalized mental health system, these centres were to be the new non-stigmatizing core of the system. To an extent, this has been the case. However, both American and the new British centres demonstrate a reluctance to offer a **total service**, that is a service for *all* of the different categories of people who experience the wide range of mental distress. In particular, centres shy away from working with people with long-term difficulties and a history of hospitalization, namely the very people now resettled in the community as part of the closure of the psychiatric hospitals (Patmore and Weaver, 1990).

While Patmore and Weaver (1991) provide useful suggestions as to how to overcome this problem, it is interesting to note that this feature of the American and British systems does not seem to have happened in Italy. If anything, most of the centres serve primarily this population. Is it therefore a cultural feature?

I would suggest that it is the outcome of the particular form the closure process took in each of these countries, and the beliefs of leading professional groups as to who they should be serving, rather than of the specific culture in which they operate.

Where closure has been approached as a positive change, mental health staff work with the continued care client as a matter of fact, and see the work with this client group as rewarding. When closure is approached as an imposed indignity, work with these services users is perceived as frustrating, beneath the 'right' level of the expertise one has been trained to provide.

This issue echoes the debate concerning 'de-professionalization' and 're-professionalization'. Are professionals to be flexible enablers, or are they to remain inflexible experts?

Day activities

The disappearance of the hospital leaves yet another empty space. People were supposed to be participating in an activity programme while in hospital, to attend a day hospital after discharge, or a day centre in the community. Day centres continue to exist. The evidence is that users prefer those centres that offer a club-like structure and in which they have a say. However, most free-of-charge places in day centres continue to be used, for the relief of informal carers and as the social refuge of the direct users.

While some day centres act as mini-institutions, others have changed dramatically in the last five years to become more like a club, and to offer opportunities to initiate and manage activities as well as to participate in ordinary community activities (Echlin, 1990). In Britain, with the growing likelihood of charging for services on the one hand and moving to a contract culture on the other, day centres may have to change even further, or disappear altogether.

Home care

For the resettled, ex 'long-stay' group of people, the group homes are the direct replacement of the hospital. It is there that the risk of re-creating mini-institutions on the one hand, and the opportunity for leading an ordinary life on the other, are at their utmost. Perring in Chapter Four and Wainwright in Chapter One have illustrated the range of possibilities for residential schemes and for the individuals who live there.

On the whole, the resettled group is happier outside the hospital, and instances of individual growth can be demonstrated, against the odds of years of hospitalization and segregation. Yet the paucity of interacting with ordinary members of the community, which Perring raised, gives cause for concern. Is the paucity due to the fears of the staff, to the assumed fears of the general public or the reluctance, or inability, of the residents?

Will it be different for a new generation that will not have the experience of long periods in psychiatric hospitals? Are group homes to be the new containment units, or the bridge between the person with the experience of mental distress and the community?

THE BID FOR NEW CONTROL MECHANISMS

The challenge of challenging behaviour

Challenging behaviour is a relatively new term, which encompasses a range of behaviours from the straightforward violent through the embarrassing (often with sexual undertones) to the withdrawn behaviour. What unites this range is that these behaviours are perceived as socially unacceptable, hidden behind the hospital's walls but exposed when the walls do not exist any more. All of a sudden there is a flurry of (mostly half-baked) discussions on challenging behaviour, as if its existence in the hospital did not matter, or as if it did not exist there.

People placed in the category of having 'challenging behaviour' are simultaneously placed also in the category of 'difficult to place', as illustrated in Chapter 1. This implies that their degree of choice of a placement in the community is considerably curtailed, they will be left in the hospital until the last moment, and they will be re-segregated with other people likewise classified.

At the same time, there is evidence to suggest that a more integrating approach, which provides specialist attention without segregation in hospital prior to resettlement and later in the community, works well in reducing the frustrations that lead to this behaviour in the first place and, secondly, in introducing alternative behaviours that are more satisfactory for the individual, society and the workers (Blunden, 1988; Ramon and Brown, 1991). Therefore, we need to ask ourselves why is this evidence not sufficiently acted upon to prevent the spread of the fear of people with challenging behaviour and the establishment of segregated units for them, either in hospitals or still existing in the community.

It would seem that 'challenging behaviour' serves a similar function to that provided by the category of 'psychopathy' at the time of its inclusion in the 1959 Mental Health Act in Britain (Ramon, 1986). Although in existence in the psychiatric literature since the 19th century, the classification of psychopathy as a separate category came about as a 'filling' of an empty space created by the abolition of the British Poor Law in 1948. Then a residual group of people who could not be easily defined either as mad or as bad or as simply poor, but which was displaying socially unacceptable behaviour, came to the fore as in need of being categorized for the sake of administrative and professional clarity — even if it was clear that no specific or new intervention has become available.

At-risk registers

At-risk or 'case' registers originated as database material in the 1960s in the Anglo Saxon world (Wing, 1984). They were hailed as providing the ultimate epidemiological data necessary for planning services.

At present, the use of these registers, and that of the new ones created in both health and social services, is changed to the identification of people assumed to be at risk due to their 'non-compliance' with the services — especially in relation to medication. Most of these people have been classified as 'the new long-stay' patients. This implies being in and out of psychiatric admissions, either in psychiatric hospitals or in psychiatric wards in general hospitals, rather than being resettled after a long stay in a psychiatric hospital.

Such registers are expected to identify these people and to focus services on them by alerting service providers to their existence. In the USA, entitlement to special programmes and financial benefits is likely to follow from such an identification, provided the client is willing to participate in the programme. As many basic benefits, food stamps among them, depend on readiness to participate in a programme, the pressure to comply increases. In Britain, such an identification is likely to lead, from 1993, to being eligible for care management assessment and intervention, being targeted for reaching out services, and for a compulsory treatment order in the community, if such an order will be agreed upon.

The advantages and disadvantages of such registers have been neatly summarized by Sayce (1991). She reflects on the contradiction between the emphasis on choice and respect in the formal services policies on the one hand and the lack of choice, the denial of access to one's file, the lack of confidentiality, and the imposition of specific types of intervention on users on the other.

I would suggest that the spread of the registers in Britain is yet another response to the closure of psychiatric hospitals, to the fear of what may happen to a vulnerable client, combined with the fear of losing control over the client yet having to account to the authorities should anything go wrong. However, those putting pressure towards establishing a register do not seem to pause and ask why do so many past service users refuse to use it. Is it simply a reflection of an illness? Could it also be a reflection of a gap between what users want and what services offer, and would we not be better off by spending more time and effort in designing services that people would like to use, rather than in attempting to control them?

Compulsory treatment in the community

Likewise, the debate around compulsory treatment in the community or the extension of guardianship orders within the existing British mental health legislation to include clinical treatment (Mental Health Act Commission, 1986) arises out of the fear of people who have been previously contained in the hospital being 'let loose'. The American, Canadian and Italian experiences of having compulsory treatment in the community (Carson, 1990; Sain *et al.*, 1990) illustrate that these can provide a beneficial framework for a small minority of people, but that informal, open access and outreach services can reach a larger group of those who have not found the formal services of much benefit.

THE RECONSIDERATION OF MAIN INTERVENTION STRATEGIES

Use, overuse, abuse and withdrawal of medication

While the psychiatric registers symbolize best the attempt to introduce new control mechanisms, it is the difficulty to enforce the regular use of medication outside the hospital that is the main motivating force behind the various forms of new controls. Many users of mental health services who complied in the hospital, usually in order to be able to leave the setting, cannot wait to stop taking medication once it is within their control. They have argued that the devastating temporary and lasting side-effects of the medication outweigh its usefulness. Especially in the community, where ordinary people are encountered, service users experience the effect of medication as disabling them from leading a more ordinary life. This applies to abilities such as concentration, crossing the road, holding down a job and making love. Yet many professionals are adamant that they should continue to take the medication, and usually for life.

Currently there are some controlled attempts to introduce self-monitoring and monitoring by informal carers, in which complaints on side-effects are taken more seriously and the degree of self-responsibility is enhanced (Birchwood *et al.*, 1989; Falloon, 1985). There are also programmes aimed at the reduction of the use of medication and the gradual withdrawal of such a use. However, the latter are discouraged by most psychiatrists, and are carried out primarily by non-medically trained people — usually in the non-profit sector or as part of a mutual support scheme of users.

At the same time, research has demonstrated the over-use of medication in psychiatric hospitals, in psychiatric wards in general hospitals and in community-based services (Muijen and Silverstone, 1987; Holloway, 1988). Furthermore, the use of multiple drugs without proven efficacy has been noted too. This widespread misuse of medication is perhaps also related to the containing function and to the felt lack of alternative interventions. Such misuse will continue to rebound on any attempt to offer users services that are helpful and not only containing.

The search for alternatives to medication has also continued. In an interesting development in Holland and Britain, attempts are made to identify positive coping styles with hearing voices and to enable others to learn and use these styles (Romme and Escher, 1991).

Psychological interventions

There is little evidence to suggest that hospital closure has led to a re-examination of most of the psychological methods of interventions used in the First World. The exception is the focus on less verbal types of counselling, utilized with people with learning and emotional difficulties, as well as with the continued care client in mental health. Promising results have been achieved by few, charismatic, therapists (Sinason, 1991; Brandon, 1990). The creation of a **life book** as a therapeutic device, which a number of homes also use, highlights the touching and most necessary attention to re-creating a life history for people who have spent so much of their life in hospital. A life book can consist of the person's old photographs, postcards of the area in which s/he grew up or lived for some time, poems and drawings that reflect their life experience in their own words, whether written by them, dictated by them or contributed by others. Some workers start a life book by giving basic information about their own life.

Try and encourage one of your clients who has a long history of hospitalization, or of moving from one placement to another, one town to another, to do a life book. See what it adds to your knowledge of the client, or what it changes in your relationships, what it adds to the person's own perception of him/herself.

Social strategies of intervention

This is a vast area, as it covers intervention from the level of a small group to that of the social structure, and is beyond the scope of this chapter. Hospital closure itself is a social strategy, as well as an administrative strategy that has implications at the level of individuals and groups.

With the closure of the psychiatric hospitals, greater focus on **networking** has taken place in several services, be they run by professionals, unqualified care staff, users or informal carers. Most of these attempts have taken place in the non-profit and social services agencies, rather than in the Health Service (Milroy, 1989; Whittaker, 1986). The development of different types of **advocacy**, mentioned in the section on citizenship, is closely related to the use of networking (Brandon, 1991). A further extension of networking is provided by the creation of **circles of support** and **brokerage** around a service user (Brandon and Towe, 1990). Good care management would also be an exercise in networking: see the scheme operated by Choice, as evaluated by Pilling (1988).

Language in transition

Changes in terminology often reflect changes in attitudes and practice. The polarization of the new terminology used in mental health services reflects the polarization in attitudes and vision currently expressed within all of those mental health systems that are in transition. Service users and those committed to their participation in the new system debate whether the right term to employ is 'users', 'consumers', 'recipients' instead of the old 'patients' and 'clients'. Some professionals, and relatives, keen on the disease model, use terms such as 'the severely mentally ill' and 'the chronically mentally ill'.

TRAINING FOR THE FUTURE

Training new workers and re-training those already working is one central route to encouraging the type of mental health system we would want to have. The major general issue concerning training for a system in transition is how to prepare practitioners to be able to approach innovation without trepidation, with due consideration, and to be able to use new ways of working in everyday practice.

An ironical observation is the fact that the more thorough the training is, the more the trained individual is committed to what s/he has been trained for, and therefore less ready for change. If anything, this state of affairs reinforces the necessity to train workers for a generalized readiness to be flexible and to have the know-how of how to handle proposed change. So far, at the level of basic training for most disciplines in mental health such a generalized readiness is not part of the training menu. The thrust of the training effort seems to go into instilling fixed ways of working, even though a range is provided and attention to individual clients is asked for. While qualifying training for a post and in-service training attempt to provide an up-dated knowledge base and how to approach, for example, policy changes, these are usually not geared to attitudinal change.

Some imaginative training schemes exist, such as:

1. The American yearly conference of all stake holders in the Community Support Schemes;
2. The PASS and PASSING group evaluation workshops with a mixed composition of stake holders (Glenn and Wolfensberger, 1983):
3. The Better Futures programme run by the King's Fund in London in which six districts across the country are given considerable support and an outside facilitator while they are re-structuring their services;
4. The requirement to prepare, run, and report on an innovation project in one's own service as part of an interdisciplinary course on mental health work with the continued care client at the London School of Economics.

Much can be learned from other fields, from private business to the introduction of technological and social change in a planned way (e.g. family planning, change in methods of agricultural production, community development projects). To ensure a lasting change it seems crucial to demystify the notion that innovation depends on considerable financial resources and can only be a 'top-down' affair. While there is a need for a 'top-down' commitment matched by resources, there is an equal need for a 'bottom-up' approach to innovation if it is to really influence everyday practice. Therefore, practitioners need to be convinced that **they** can do it, and **how** to go about it.

Each chapter in this book contains several examples of small-scale innovations that indicate some of the necessary steps to be taken to ensure the success of an attempt to innovate. In Chapter Three, the section on 'The conceptual and moral underpinning of the planned closure' has outlined the necessary conditions for innovation.

VISION

The **content** of the desirable training depends on the type of system we would like. Across the book, and in particular in Chapter 3, the type of knowledge and skills that a participative mental health system requires have been outlined.

Do we need an overall vision? Vision can be a derided word in a pragmatic world, used for lip-service purposes, covering for lack of genuine intention and knowledge. Yet it can also be about focusing on the type of system/world we would like to have and lead to steps taken towards reaching the ideal.

While the text has illustrated the existence of individuals and small teams looking for a vision and struggling towards it, it also demonstrated the lack of an overall vision for the British mental health system, including the closure component. I would argue that both the American and the Italian systems have had an overall vision, and have benefited from it, despite all of the many shortcomings which each of these systems has.

The American vision of mental health centres as replacements of the psychiatric hospitals in 1963, and of the Community Support System since the 1970s (Stroul, 1982) has led to considerable achievements in providing a varied, good quality service and greater participation among the different stake holders. Both visions have also provided yardsticks against which to measure the state-of-the-art of existing services, and the possibility of wide-ranging experimentation. The American social system, rather than its mental health system, has also led to the creation of a strong voice of service users, and to innovation in user-managed services.

The Italian vision of dismantling psychiatric hospitals as social institutions of segregation, or ensuring the visibility of people with mental illness in our midst and of treating them as people with ordinary problems, has led to a heightened professional and public interest and awareness of the experience of institutionalization and of mental illness. Besides demonstrating that a reasonable mental health system can exist without psychiatric hospitals, it has also led to the establishment of generic mental health centres. In addition there has been considerable change in the role of professionals and more genuine interdisciplinary work, as well as greater participation of the politicians and interested members of the general public in decision-making concerning the services.

So far, Britain has been lagging behind these two societies in lacking an overall vision, despite a renowned tradition of social psychiatry. The emerging new participants and the changes we are now witnessing in the British mental health system could, and should, provide the impetus for the new visions, even though these may be contradictory. The task of creating a vision does not belong to one group only; it is up to each individual and each group to consider the ideal that is worth striving towards, even if it is never reached, and even if one may be branded 'utopian' for daring to declare a vision.

Not forgetting that the vision is only the first step is equally important, as is the readiness to modify the focus of the vision in the light of real changes, rather than treat it as a dogma. However, between modifying the vision and the prevailing pragmatism, which hides not only the lack of vision but the clinging to an obsolete vision, there is a world of difference.

Having indulged in preaching to you, let me make a pragmatic suggestion:

Try out the following (modified from Basset and Brunning, 1989).

1. *Let each member of the group represent a different stake holder in the mental health system.*
2. *Let them discuss and reach an agreement as to how to position themselves in relation to the others in a group sculpture.*
3. *Let them experience the physical position and the sensations it brings with it.*
4. *Let them discuss and reach an agreement as to the noise (no recognized words are allowed) that suits their position in the sculpture.*
5. *Let them make the noise, all of them together, then each of them separately, while the others are listening.*

If you and your group have experienced chaos and yet you were able to turn it into a meaningful message, then this is a positive sign that you are on your way to listening to other stake holders and to yourself, as well as being listened to, and on your way to freeing yourself from the rigid hold of past traditions, without having to discard all that was good in these traditions.

REFERENCES

Bassett, T. and Brunning, H. (1989) *Power Stations: A Workshop Exploring the Issue of Power in Multidisciplinary Teams*. Pavilion Publishing, Brighton.

Birchwood, M., Smith, J. and Macmillan, F. (1989) Predicting relapse in schizophrenia: the development and implementation of an early signs monitoring system using patients and families as observers, a preliminary investigation. *Psychological Medicine*, **19**, 649–656.

Blunden, R. (1988) *Working with People with Challenging Behaviour*. King's Fund Publications, London.

Brandon, D. (1990) *Ordinary Magic*. Tao, Preston.

Brandon, D. (1991) *Innovation Without Change?* Macmillan, London, pp. 116–42.

Brandon, D. and Towe, N. (1990) *Free to Choose*. Good Impressions, London.

Carrier, J. (1990) Sociopolitical influences on mental health care policy in the United Kingdom. In: Marks, I. and Scott, R. (eds) *Mental Health Care Delivery: Innovations, Impediments and Implementation*. Cambridge University Press, Cambridge, pp. 118–36.

Carson, D. (ed.) (1990) *Risk-taking in Mental Disorder*. Lontec, New Jersey.

Dell'Aqcua, G. and Mezzina, R. (1991) Approaching mental distress. In: Ramon, S. (ed.) *Psychiatry in Transition*. Pluto Press, London.

De Nicola, P., Giacobi, E. and Rogialli, S. (1991) Changing professional roles in the Italian psychiatric system. In: Ramon, S. (ed.) *Psychiatry in Transition*. Pluto Press, London.

Echlin, R. (ed.) (1990) *Day Care Pack*. Good Practices in Mental Health, London.

Echlin, R. and Ramon, S. (1992) Safe as houses, *Nursing Times, January 15th, 38–41*.

Falloon, I. (1985) *Family Management of Schizophrenia*. Johns Hopkins University Press, Baltimore.

Glenn, T. and Wolfensberger, W. (1983) *Program Analysis of Service Systems: Implementation of Normalization Goals (PASSING), Normalization Criteria and Rating Manual*, 2nd ed. Canadian Institute of Mental Retardation, Toronto.

Henelly, R. (1991) Mental Health Resource Centres. In: Ramon, S. (ed.) *Psychiatry in Transition*. Pluto Press, London.

Holloway, F. (1988) Prescribing for the long-term mentally ill: a study of treatment practice, *British Journal of Psychiatry*, **149**, 75–81.

Jones, K. and Poletti, A. (1985) Understanding the Italian experience, *British Journal of Psychiatry*, **146**, 341–7.

Mental Health Act Commission (1986) *Compulsory Treatment in the Community: A Discussion Paper*. See also the proposal by the Royal College of Psychiatrists (1987) Community Treatment Orders, June.

Milroy, A. (1989) Changing our professional ways. In: Brackx, A. and Grimshaw C. (eds.) *Mental Health Care in Crisis*, Pluto Press, London.

Mitchell, R. (1990) The Barnet Intensive Crisis Intervention Team. In: Cohen G. and Ramon, S. (eds.) *The Role of Social Workers in the 1983 Mental Health Act: Innovations in Practice*. BASW Publications, Birmingham.

Muijen, M. and Silverstone, T. (1987) A comparative hospital survey of psychotropic drug prescribing, *British Journal of Psychiatry*, **150**, 501–4.

Patmore, C. and Weaver, T. (1990) Rafts on an open sea. *Health Service Journal*, 27–32.

Patmore, C. and Weaver, T. (1991) *Community Mental Health Teams: Lessons for Planners and Managers.* Good Practices in Mental Health, London.

Pilling, D. (1988) *The Case Manager Project: Summary of the Evaluation Project.* Rehabilitation Resource Centre, City University, London.

Ramon, S. (1986) The category of psychopathy in British Law. In: Miller, P. and Rose, N. (eds.) *The Power of Psychiatry.* Polity Press, Oxford.

Ramon, S. (1989) The reactions of English-speaking professionals to the Italian psychiatric reform, *International Journal of Social Psychiatry*, **35 (1)**, 120–8.

Ramon, S. and Brown, M. (1991) The challenge of challenging behaviour, *Community Care*, **861**, 16–17.

Romme, M. and Escher, S. (1991) Heard but not seen, *Openmind*, **49**, 20–2.

Sain, F., Norcio, B. and Malannino, S. (1990) Compulsory health treatment: the experience in Trieste from 1978 to 1988, *Mental Health*, **4**, 137–52.

Savio, M. (1991) Psychiatric nursing in Italy: an extinguished profession or an emerging professionalism? *International Journal of Social Psychiatry*, **39**, 293–9.

Sayce, L. (1991) Registering — a risky business, *Social Work Today*, **22**, 14–16.

Sinason, V. (1991) *The Sense in Stupidity: Mental Handicap and Psychotherapy.* Free Association, London.

Stroul, B. (1982) *Community Support Program.* Analysis of State Strategies, Boston University Centre for Rehabilitation Research and Training in Mental Health, 730 Commonwealth Avenue, Boston, MA, 02770.

Turner, B.S. (1990) Outline of a theory of citizenship, *Sociology*, **24**, 2.

Youll, P. and Perring, C. (1991) *Consumer Approaches in Residential Care.* Seminar held in Brunel University, Uxbridge, May 25th.

Yuval-Davis, N. (1991) Women, the State and Ethnic Processes — the citizenship debate, *Critical Social Policy* **31**, 46–62.

Warner, R. (1991) Building creative programmes, In: Ramon, S. (ed.) *Beyond Community Care: Normalization and Integration Work.* Macmillan, London.

Whittaker, J. K. (1986) Integrating formal and informal care: a conceptual framework. *British Journal of Social Work*, Suppl., **16**, 39–62.

Wing, J. K. (1984) *Report of the Camberwell Register*, 1964–1984, MRC Social Psychiatry Unit, Institute of Psychiatry, London.

Appendix A: The British context

The majority of mental health services are offered by the statutory sector, followed by the voluntary sector (Table 1). To date, the commercial sector provides relatively few services, and is concentrated in the provision of individual specialist consultation, housing and a small number of hospitals

Table A1. The structure of mental health services in Britain[a]

Statutory sector	Voluntary	Commercial
Primary care (NHS)	Welfare advice Legal advice	Private p.c.
Specialist out-patients service (psychiatrists, psychologists, ot, CPNs) (NHS)	Self-help	Private Specialists
Social Services		
MH teams (PSS)		
Income support (SS through PSS)		
Mental health centres (multi- or uni-disciplinary (NHS and PSS)	Drop-in centres MH centres (ethnic minorities)	
Crisis service (NHS, PSS)		
Home treatment (NHS) Psychiatric wards in general hospital (NHS)	Beginnings of sanctuaries	
Psychiatric hospital (NHS) (PSS -sw input)		Psychiatric hospitals
Sheltered housing (PSS)	Housing	Housing
Day care (NHS and Social Services)	Day care	
Employment schemes (PSS) Resettlement teams (PSS)	Employment schemes	
Users' groups	Users' groups	
Relatives' groups (PSS)	Relatives' groups	
Outreach projects (PSS and NHS)	Outreach projects Pressure groups	

[a]NHS: National Health Service; PSS; Personal Social Services

(which cater either for people with minor mental health problems or those with extremely severe difficulties). However, the table does not tell us about the availability, accessibility, content, quality and variability of these services across the country.

At present (1991) there are 110 Psychiatric Hospitals in the UK, with 190 510 admissions in 1987–8 in England (i.e. excluding Scotland and Wales). (This number for admissions should not be confused with the number of people admitted, as some people have been admitted more than once.) There are also psychiatric beds in general hospitals. Out of all admissions, 63% do not last for more than one month and a further 24% are completed within a month (HPSSS, 1990).

Some of the basic social inequalities are reflected in these statistics, namely that proportionally more women and more members of the Afro-Caribbean ethnic minority are admitted across all categories of admission. Of particular concern is the finding that Afro-Caribbean young men are admitted to hospital through the initiative of the police (Rogers and Faulkner, 1987; Barnes *et al.*, 1990; Bean *et al.* 1991), as this may reflect on the use of admission to deflect assumed but unproven aggression. The more general issue of services meeting the needs and wishes of women and of ethnic minorities will be looked at in the concluding section of the book.

There were 1 603 300 out-patient appointments in 1989–9, and 41 000 Day Hospital attenders. Thus the majority of the British population with mental health problems live outside hospitals for most of the time. Nevertheless two-thirds of the NHS mental health budget (about two billion pounds) is spent on hospitals, and only 2.5% of the personal social services departments is spent directly on mental health services (HPSSS, 1990).

Furthermore, although the number of mental health centres has increased considerably in the last five years, from 20 in 1986 to 150 in 1990 (Sayce, 1990), there are only 150 such centres in the whole country. This provides a rough indication as to the continuing gap between an over-developed hospital sector and an under-developed community service sector.

THE POLICY CONTEXT

Although hospital closure was mentioned in 1963 by Mr E. Powell, the then Minister of Health, as part of the future vision, it was not until 1975 that the Ministry decided to fund one pilot project of such a closure. This has become known as the Worcester project (Hall, 1990). It took between 1975 and 1989 to resettle all of the 198 residents of two hospitals (St Wulstan and Powick) into alternative settings, even though new admissions to these hospitals stopped in 1978; this compared with 1000 residents resettled over ten years in Trieste, or 3000 in Turin over a similar period (Del Giudice *et al.*, 1991; Pirella, 1987). The new settings consisted of sheltered accommodation (primarily hostels), rehabilitation units, day care (in day hospitals and day centres), a new psychogeriatric unit, and an acute intervention unit in the general hospital. A considerable increase in home visiting by nurses took place. The accompanying evaluation has illustrated that ex-patients were satisfied with the change, as were the local GPs. Surprisingly no community mental health centres, or multidisciplinary teams, seem to have been planned as part of the alternatives to hospital care.

Although the Worcester project was researched, the research component did not look at the staff's perspective, that of the community, or the relatives. No mention of the process of closure beyond the different stages has been made, and only the cost of the new services is mentioned, without the calculation of what it would cost to continue with the psychiatric hospital as the core of the services. It remains unclear why it took 14 years to close the two, rather small, hospitals. Tellingly, at the conference convened to mark the final closure this issue was not even raised. Ex-patients were not invited to present their experience of leaving the hospital and their new life in the community. Likewise the voluntary sector was not mentioned. The whole project seems to have been conducted with the intent to supplement hospitalization, rather than search and establish for alternatives to it.

In 1982, the then Minister of Health, Mr N. Fowler, announced that the Government was calling on Regional Health Authorities to decide and plan the closure of large psychiatric hospitals. It was recognized that this would require additional financial resources — especially in the period in which hospital services would continue to operate while those in the community were being established. Joint funding between the health and social services, and later a 'dowry' system of financing the resettlement of individual long-term residents of the psychiatric hospitals, was made available to meet these needs. The debate as to the feasibility of the funding system, the strings attached, and whether the sums included were/are sufficient continues. An indication of the degree of variability of funding available in different parts of the country is provided by the range of 'dowry' sums, from £11 000 to £22 000 per person.

It was also assumed that Health Authorities would sell closed hospitals sites and re-use the income in community services. With the current slump in the value of such sites, several authorities have been unable to do so, thus closure plans were curtailed accordingly. Nevertheless, from 1991, Health Authorities have to pay a capital tax on buildings that they own. This is assumed to establish a 'dis-incentive' to own buildings.

To date, the closure programmes relate only to people who have been in hospital for more than two years, the so-called 'long-stay' patients, and not to the majority that enters psychiatric hospitals for a short period (the 'acute' patients), even though it is well known that many in this group return to hospital for subsequent admissions and constitute a high-risk group and are likely to become long-term users of mental health services.

It would therefore seem that the Government intended to encourage the closure of large psychiatric hospitals, rather than that of all hospitals, and/or a restructure of the mental health system. As a direct result of the Government's pressure, 40 hospitals have been earmarked for closure throughout England and Wales, and none in Scotland. Out of these 40 hospitals, only five have already closed. Of the three hospitals described in detail in this book, two are due for their final closure within 12–18 months. It seems unlikely now that the third hospital will close down, even though it is already half empty. Formally the Regional Health Authority argues that it has run out of the money with which to finance the final closure; opposition of senior clinical staff must have contributed to this state of affairs. The situation in the other hospitals due for closure varies too, from those about to close, those in the process and those unlikely to close even though the process began a few years ago. Thus, although each of the hospitals in our study has unique features, the process they share has more similarities than is usually acknowledged by those involved in it.

THE LEGISLATIVE CONTEXT

The closure of psychiatric hospitals does not form a part of the British legislation concerning health and welfare. Likewise, the structure of the mental health services in the community is left to the understanding of each Health District and Social Services department. This state of affairs contrasts with the American legislation on mental health centres in 1963 and the right to treatment in 1980, as well as with the Italian 1978 legislation, which allowed the closure of hospitals and the establishment of mental health centres.

There are advantages and disadvantages to an unlegislated system. We need to ask ourselves whether a changing system is helped or hindered by legislation that takes on board the desired direction of change. Legislation provides a stamp of approval and a reinforcement of specific directions, and can prevent or limit the development of other directions. In this case, legislation could potentially encourage or discourage the closure of hospitals, the creation of comprehensive services in the community, limit or enhance the power of any of the stake holders in the field of mental health (e.g. administrators, professionals, unqualified care staff, service users, relatives or the general public). There has been no professional or public pressure to legislate in full the change of the mental health service system, but there has been a recent attempt to legislate the right to assessment and a planned package of care prior to discharge. This now forms a part of the new NHS and Community Care Act of 1990, and has been included at the insistence of the relatives, pressure group (the National Schizophrenia Fellowship, NSF) and its supporters in the House of Lords and the House of Commons. It is most doubtful whether this piece of legislation would lead to fundamental changes, as the law is unspecific as to the nature of the assessment, care package, and whose responsibility it is to see the package through and resource it.

The NHS and Community Care Act 1990

Although compulsory entry to hospitalization is legislated in the Mental Health Act 1959 and the Amendments of 1983, the 1990 Act is of greater relevance to 95% of the long-term users of the mental health services, as only 5% are the subject of a compulsory admission. The main components of the act concern:

Purchasing and service provision

Purchasing and providing services in the NHS are to be separate units within each Health Authority. This split is hailed by some as the most important opportunity for the purchasers to establish new mental health services, and by others as a recipe for chaos and a money-only led service.

NHS units as autonomous trusts

Units in the NHS can become autonomous trusts, which have the right to capital revenues, the right to decide on pay to its employees, the right to refuse or offer health intervention to people who live in the catchment area. It is unclear what, if any, obligations they have to the Health District that has established them in the first place.

Trusts are seen by some as a flexible innovation that will benefit all of us and by others as a fragmenting device aimed at the near future privatization of the NHS.

GP budgets

GPs can have their own budget, within which they are free to buy services as they choose, but neither have the obligation to explain to their patients the reasons for their decisions, nor to offer equitable treatment to all patients. Until now, GPs could refer people to any specialist treatment, which was also financed by the NHS, and did not have to pay for it. GPs who would not become budget holders are afraid of being given a less preferential treatment within the NHS than those with such a budget.

Quality assurance mechanisms

Quality assurance mechanisms are to be introduced, which will include not only quality assurance officers (already in existing in Health Districts for the last two years) but also the need to consult service users in the evaluation of services, the need to establish a complaints procedure and autonomous inspection units. No one doubts the usefulness of such measures or the justification of emphasizing quality assurance. There are, however, serious doubts as to whether resources necessary for establishing these mechanisms will become available (especially to local authorities) and whether users' views will be taken on board after being collected, as well as how thorough will be the effort to consult users.

Local authority co-ordination

Local authorities are to have a lead role in the co-ordination of community care for people with disabilities, including mental distress. While this has been seen as finally accepting that community care is primarily about social care, rather than medical care, there are doubts as to the ability of Local Authorities' services as they are now to provide this care, and whether the resources will become available when the law will be fully implemented. A complicated formula for the resources per capita has appeared in the White Paper (*Caring for People*, 1988) that led to the legislation and which made it clear that Central Government had no intention of covering the cost in full. It is therefore unclear where the rest of the necessary funding will come from, how easy will be the transfer of resources from the Health Service to the Social Services, and if indeed such transfer is to take place or whether we are likely to see an amalgamation of health and social services in this field proposed in the near future.

Furthermore, although put in the lead role, Local Authorities are instructed to become enablers and overseers rather than direct providers of services.

Individual assessment and care packages

People with a disability will have the right to assessment, and to the co-ordination of their individualized care package (known as 'care management'). However, the following remains unclear: (a) whether every person with a disability will have this right, or only those with a serious disability; (b) who will decide; (c) what redress will exist regarding such decisions; (d) who will be the care managers; and (e) whether they will have a devolved budget or not. Several care management projects have been piloted in Britain since the early 1980s, most of which focused on people with physical disability (Chesterman *et al.*, 1988). A pilot project focused on mental health service users is currently implemented in five districts and is co-ordinated by Research and Development in Psychiatry (RDP). All of these projects have been sponsored by the Department of Health.

The American experience has been variable, and it would seem that everything can take place under the name of care management (Beardshaw and Towell, 1990).

The mental health specific grant

For the first time in the history of the mental health services in Britain, a small amount of money has been 'ring-fenced' for the purpose of establishing innovations in this field, no doubt in recognition of the level of need to do so. The sums involved are very small (currently £20 million for the whole country — roughly £120 000 for a county). Projects are run by Local Authorities in agreement with the Health Authorities as from April 1991, and are closely monitored by the Social Services Inspectorate (SSI).

So far it has been heartening to observe the high degree of interest and commitment that this grant has generated, as well as the wide range of initiatives proposed (e.g. mental health services for ethnic minorities, user-run services, alternatives to hospitalization, crisis services, respite care, mental health resource centres). It is too early to know whether the grant will indeed generate the width and depth of innovation that is required for the transformation of the mental health services from a hospital-based core to a community-based core, or not.

While the NHS part of the Act has already been applied since April 1991, only the mental health specific grant has been implemented out of the Community Care component of the Act. The rest of this element is to be implemented only from April 1993, raising doubts concerning the degree of political commitment to this part of the Act.

THE EMERGING PARTNERS IN THE BRITISH SCENE

Service users

During the 1980s, we have witnessed the considerable growth of user groups and user involvement in Britain, analysed by Rogers and Pilgrim (1991). In particular, the voluntary sector (with Mind in the lead role) has taken on board this involvement, encouraging the development of users' participation. Up to now social services trailed behind the voluntary sector, with some interesting and innovative initiatives (Hennelly, 1991). The Health Service seemed to have ignored this development until the application of the NHS part of the 1990 NHS and Community Care Act. Presently there are several examples of new initiatives taken by Health and Social Services authorities to utilize existing users' groups and encourage the formation of new ones, especially as partners to planning and evaluation (Barker, 1991; Perring, 1991). 'Top-down' and 'bottom-up' approaches can be discerned (Somekh, 1991). The cynics would doubt how genuine all of this is, arguing that only when power is divested from the formal authorities and the professionals to the users will this move be more than tokenistic.

Relatives

This group too has come to the fore in the 1980s much more than before. The NSF, the only well known relatives' organization, has more than 6000 members. Social services and Mind also have relatives' groups attached to local branches, which provide some support.

The NSF has campaigned publicly against the closure of the psychiatric hospitals, together with another pressure group, SANE (Schizophrenia Emergency Campaign). Although the latter has attempted to frighten the general public by a publicity campaign that portrayed people with schizophrenia as dangerous and menacing, there are no signs that the public has accepted these views. While the national newspapers and television continue to portray mostly the failures of community care, rather than its successes in relation to people with mental illness, the general public seems to assume that hospital closure is a reasonable step towards well-resourced community services, and would like the Government to invest more in these services (McKie, 1990). Thus at the political level and that of the general public relatives may get a sympathetic ear, although this does not seem to apply to policy decisions, unlike the situation in the USA.

Care staff

Although the number of care staff has increased considerably in Britain in the last decade as a direct result of hospital closure, the care staff are not a coherent, cohesive or 'heard' group. As suggested in the Introduction, this reflects on its internal and external ambiguous, almost marginalized, position. This, in turn, mirrors the process of **being in change**, which is where British society is *vis-a-vis* mental health issues, and people who suffer from mental illness.

The non-statutory sector

This sector has expanded considerably during the 1980s as a service provider, as a direct result of the Government's encouragement. The latter attempted to cut down the statutory sector and replace it by non-profit (voluntary) and for-profit services.

However, while the for-profit sector has expanded primarily in housing provision, the non-profit services have expanded in all directions. This has been the case because there is no profit to be made from most other services in the field of mental illness, with some exceptions such as consultations and hospitalization for people with private health insurance who, for the time being, are a minority in the population.

Yet, paradoxically, the continuation of the expansion of this sector is threatened by the same government that has enticed them to expand. Under the new regulations, the cost of housing is not fully covered by Central Government through its social security arm. Instead, the Government expects Local Authorities and/or relatives to top up any additions incurred due to inflation, in its attempt to cut down the expenditure on housing. As housing has been the most lucrative area for for-profit agencies, it is likely that a number of them will disappear from an insecure market. This latest twist illustrates nicely the degree of reliability of the for-profit subsector as a service provider for people with mental illness.

The non-profit organizations now face a new challenge with the split in purchasing and provision in the NHS and the move to a contract culture in both the NHS and the social services with the introduction of care management programmes. Central Government has also attempted to curtail the campaigning role of the non-profit organizations, arguing that their charitable status excludes campaigning. Such an attempt goes against the grain of the long-honoured tradition of the British non-profit sector, as well as against the interests of the people represented by these organizations.

REFERENCES

Barker, I. (1991) *User Views in Purchasing and Contracts*. Conference on Effective Consumer Feedback in Mental Health Services, 11th–12th June, RDP, London.
Barnes, M., Bowl, R. and Fisher, M. (1990) *Sectioned: Social Services and the 1983 Mental Health Act*. Routledge, London.
Bean, P., Bingley, W., Bynore, I., Faulkner, A., Rassaby, E. and Rogers, A. (1991) *Out of Harm's Way*. Mind Publications, London.
Beardshaw, V. and Towell, D. (1990) *Case Management*. King's Fund Publications, London.
Chesterman, J., Challis, D. and Davies, B. (1988) Long-term care at home for the elderly: a four-year follow-up, *British Journal of Social Work*, **18** (Suppl), 43–53.
Del Giudice, G., Evaristo, P. and Reali, M. (1991) How can Mental Hospitals be Phased Out? In: Ramon, S. (ed.) *Psychiatry in Transition*. Pluto Press, London.
Hall, P. (1990) Closure of the Worcestershire asylums and their replacement by a new community-based service. In: Hall, P. and Brockington, I. (eds.) *The Closure of Mental Hospitals*. Gaskell, London.
Hennelly, R. (1991) Mental health resource centres. In: Ramon, S. (ed.) *Psychiatry in Transition*. Pluto Press, London.
Health and Personal Social Services Statistics (1990). HMSO, London.
McKie, D. (1990) Mentally Ill Aid Doubted, *The Guardian*, July 23rd.
Perring, C. (1991) *Issues from Consumer-Oriented Research, Caring in Homes Initiative*, Department of Government, Brunel University, Uxbridge.
Pirella, A. (1987) The implementation of the Italian psychiatric reform in a large conurbation, *International Journal of Social Psychiatry*, **33(2)**, 119-31.
Rogers, A. and Faulkner, A. (1987) *A Place of Safety*. Mind Publications, London.
Rogers, A. and Pilgrim, D. (1991) 'Pulling down churches': accounting for the British mental health users' movement, *Sociology of Health and Illness*, **13(2)**, 129–47.
Sayce, L. (1990) *Community Mental Health Services in Britain: The Pace of Development*. Research and Development in Psychiatry, London.
Somekh, D. (1991) A District Strategy. Conference on Effective Consumer Feedback in Mental Health Services, 11th–12th June, RDP, London.

Index

Italy
  professional reactions to closures
    99–101

Job satisfaction, in mental health work
  94

Knowledge, professional   86–7

Labelling theory   125–6
Leave-taking   147–8
Legislation   109, 187–90
Life book   178
Life histories   164
Living accommodation, normalization
    62–4
Local authorities, and coordination of
    community care   188
Loss, and change   145–7

Management committees, users as
    members   xxiii
Medication
  in group homes   158
  use and misuse   177–8
Mental health professionals, sources of
    ambiguity and ambivalence
    91–6
Mental health specific grant   189
Mental health work
  attractions of   92–3
  interdisciplinary   94–6
  job satisfaction   94
  and risk-taking   93
Mental illness, as a social role   124–6
Mutual help groups   xxiii

National Health Service, reorganizations
    53–4
Neighbours, informing   37
Networking   178
NHS and Community Care Act 1990   109,
    188–90
NHS trusts   188
Non-compliant clients   xvi
Non-profit agencies, *see* Voluntary
    organizations
Non-statutory sector   xxiv–xxv, 191

Normalization   xvii, xix–xxii, 13, 21,
    60–1, 127–8
  criticisms of   xxii
  elements   59–60
  in living accommodation   62–4
  passing system   60–2
North East Thames RHA, closure policy
    50–1
  challenge of   55–6
  and community placements   56–7
  conflicts arising   64–81
  humanity   54–5
  motivation   53–4
  reaffirmation of chronicity   57–9
NSF   190
Nursing
  as a semi-profession   87
  students failing to complete training
    89
Nursing staff
  conflicts arising out of closure policies
    65–6
  defence mechanisms   89–90
  involvement   79–80
  reservations about closures   66–7
  responses to closures   99–101
  training   137

Occupational therapy, as a semi-
    profession   87
Open Door policy   xiv

Para-professionals   91
Participative model   169–71
Partners, emerging   xxii–xxv
Patients
  assessment   32–4, 138–42
  direct contact with   134–5
  lack of choice   135
  lack of facilities for self-care   136
  lack of privacy   135
  preparation for leaving hospital
    136–8
  selection for placement in houses
    35–6, 142–3, 163–4
  view of ward life   132–4
  visits to group homes   144–5
  see also Residents; Users